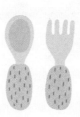

All-Organic
Baby Food Cookbook

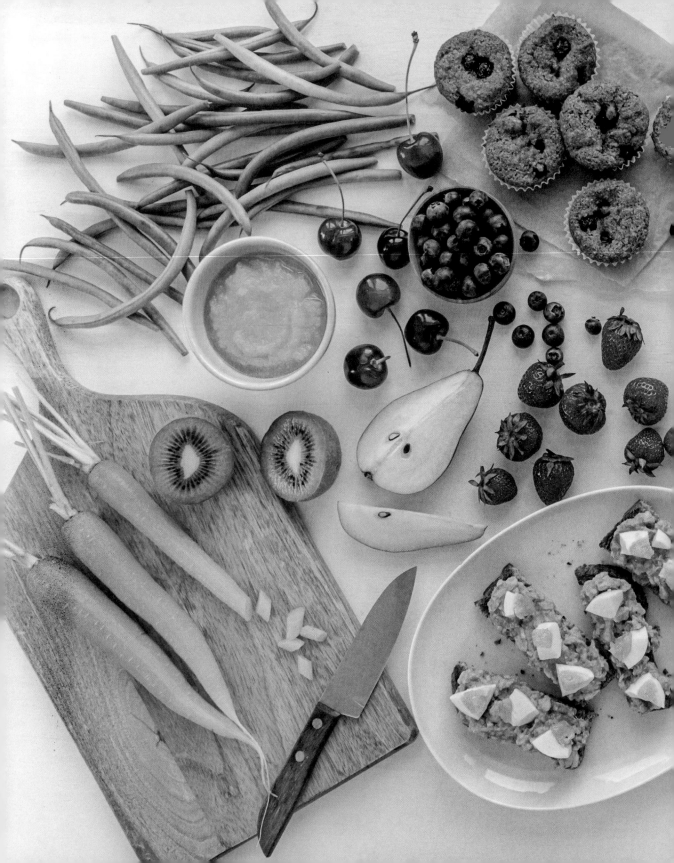

All-Organic Baby Food

COOKBOOK

FIRST-TIME PARENT'S GUIDE TO NUTRITIOUS FOODS FOR EVERY AGE & STAGE

LEAH BODENBACH, RN, BSN

Photography by Nancy Cho

ZEITGEIST · NEW YORK

Copyright © 2020 by Penguin Random House LLC

Published in the United States by Zeitgeist, an imprint of Zeitgeist™, a division of Penguin Random House LLC, New York.

penguinrandomhouse.com

Zeitgeist™ is a trademark of Penguin Random House LLC

ISBN: 9780593196755
Ebook ISBN: 9780593196762

Photography by Nancy Cho
Illustrations by Kateryna Kovalova
Book design by Katy Brown

Printed in the United States of America

1 3 5 7 9 10 8 6 4 2

First Edition

For Elowen and Aldrik
& for every child:
May your little bodies be nourished
and strong as you grow. May you impact future
generations and lead the way in health.

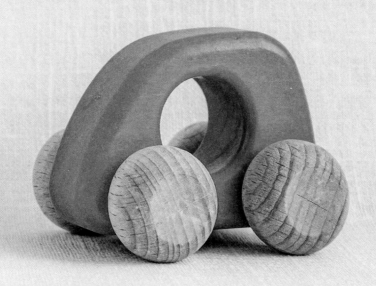

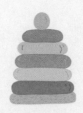

Contents

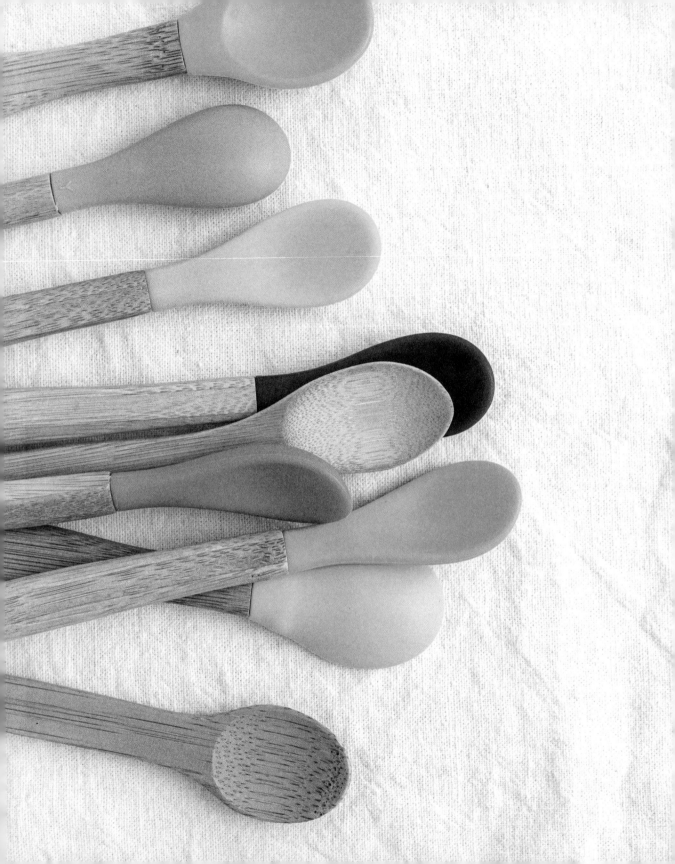

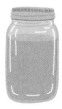

Introduction

Welcome to one of the most important transitions in being a new parent: feeding your baby solids! As with any new milestone in your baby's life, you probably have a lot of questions: *How can I best nourish my little one? Do I always have to buy organic? What's the difference between a food sensitivity and a food allergy?* As a holistic health coach with a background in pediatric nursing, I have worked with many parents in your shoes, answering questions like these and helping them navigate all the choices (and pressures!) in feeding first foods.

As a mother, I also know just how overwhelming it can be trying to figure out what's best for your child. After my first baby was born, I thought, *This won't be too hard. I take care of babies for a living.* I thought my experience as a pediatric, labor and delivery, and postpartum nurse would make things come naturally to me. While some things did come naturally, like snuggling with my baby, posting pictures of us at the park, and kissing her cute, tiny nose, other things were not as smooth, like figuring out how to get rid of her chronic diaper rash and eczema. We changed our laundry soap, tried multiple clean brands of diapers and wipes, and tested natural zinc oxide cream, organic baby powder, antifungal cream, as well as natural remedies and salves. What we *hadn't* been paying attention to was the foods she and I were eating. It turned out she had an underlying egg allergy that was presenting itself as chronic diaper rash and eczema.

This discovery made even more sense once I learned that food allergies, chronic illnesses, mental illness, and eczema (among other things) had one thing in common: an unhealthy gut. I then became wildly passionate about reshaping my own gut health and nurturing hers. I learned that the combination of your gut microbiome, genetic predisposition, and toxin exposure can trigger chronic illnesses like allergies or autoimmune disorders. These discoveries ignited my path toward becoming a nurse coach for mothers and babies, as I began to integrate my knowledge in scientific and medical research with a holistic approach.

As parents, we possess great powers to help foster the growth of a healthy baby, starting with nourishing foods and low-toxin living. We might not get a say in our genetics, or some of our toxin exposures, but we get a big say in foods, starting with our baby's first bites. One of the best benefits to making your own homemade baby food is that you get to know each and every ingredient your baby is eating!

In this book, I'll walk you through your baby's nutritional needs from about six months old to toddlerhood. Chapter 1 introduces you to organic foods, including how to shop organic on a budget and navigate the farmer's market and the grocery aisles for the freshest foods. Chapters 2 and 3 explore your baby's gut, nutrient needs, first foods, how to cook for your baby with minimal equipment, and even care for yourself during this time as a parent. Chapter 4 delves into food allergies and intolerances, how to introduce foods, and foods to avoid during the first year. This chapter also reveals why bone broth is one of the most important first foods. Finally, chapters 5 through 9 are filled with recipes that start with the first bite, all the way to great toddler snacks and family meals!

The core nutritional guideline I carry throughout the book focuses on a balance of essential nutrients, healthy fats, and good gut bacteria to help support the demands of a growing baby. I offer recommendations throughout, along with 125 recipes, but ultimately you get to choose what makes the most sense for your family. I encourage you to move out of your comfort zone and

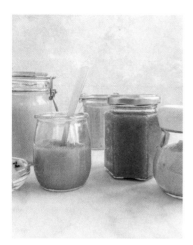 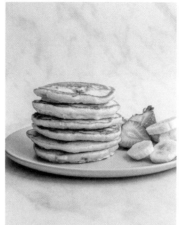 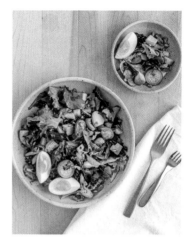

give your baby brain-boosting, nutrient-dense foods you might not like or haven't tried yet—you may both learn something new and delicious along the way.

When we supply our children with the essential nutrients from food, we give them the opportunity to achieve their full potential in every way. Serving whole foods is one of the most protective ways we can provide for their little bodies. If you're wondering about how much money or time this might take, I'll provide you with helpful tips to make decisions about buying organic and how to make the most of your organic dollar. Also, all the recipes in this book are meant to be easy. You can make trays of homemade baby food (and freeze for later use) or create family-friendly meals in an hour or less. This will allow you to enjoy more time living, without compromising your food choices and quality.

With everything that comes with being a first-time parent, my hope is that this book will make introducing solids fun and easy, while helping you take charge of your entire family's health. I'm honored to be a part of this important milestone in your child's life and food journey. Let's dig in!

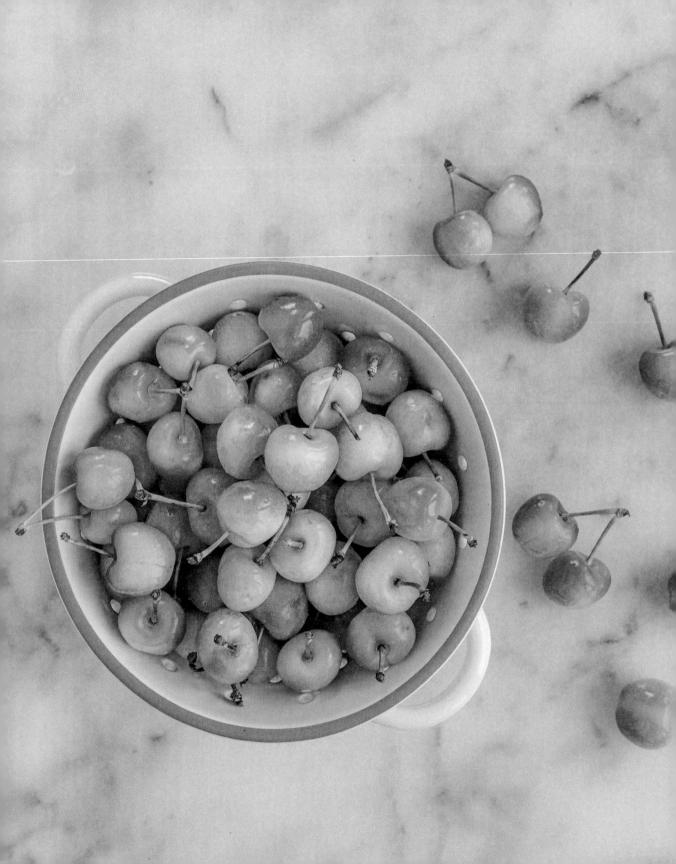

One
A Clean, Organic Start

What does it mean to eat organic, especially for babies? This chapter answers that question, along with how to eat organic on a budget, choose the cleanest foods, and select the best version of food varieties such as meat, vegetables, and fruits.

Eating the Rainbow

Healthy eating means buying the best foods we can with the resources we have. That means feeding our babies organic, in-season, local foods across the colors of the rainbow as much as possible, so that they eat foods with the most abundant and varied nutrients. Healthy eating doesn't have to be limited to organic food either; it can also mean buying non-organic produce and simply washing them well (see page 34). As different types of food contain a variety of nutritional benefits, the more diversity we include in meals, the stronger our immune systems and minds can become. Offering little ones lots of fruits, vegetables, good fats, and good proteins is one of the greatest things we can do for them (see Resources, page 234 for more on eating the rainbow).

In addition to a rainbow of color, you'll want to introduce and serve a rainbow of textures, flavors, and food groups. This will set the stage for your baby to continue to be open and flexible to trying new foods. Studies have shown that the greater the variety of flavors introduced before age one, and *continuously* offered beyond the first year, the more likely children are to keep trying and enjoying different flavors. For example, fish might be a weird flavor for kids if they hadn't eaten it before age one. Same with meats. Too often, parents say their children won't eat meat or fish, but if we look at their child's diet between ages six months and two years, it often shows that they didn't have a lot of repeat exposures to these foods. Some parents may do a really good job varying fruits and vegetables, but may not be as diligent in introducing different kinds of meat or fish. Ideally, you'll want to begin broadening your child's palate before age one and then continue it through their first years and beyond.

Going Organic

Organic food is best for babies because pesticide exposure can contribute to a number of health problems. For example, the endocrine system (the body system in charge of hormone production) can be overworked if it accumulates toxins. Since babies have much smaller bodies, it means toxins can accumulate in higher amounts for them. When the body has fewer toxins to work against, it can function at its highest level: immunity-wise, developmentally, and physically.

It's also more environmentally friendly to eat locally and organically, as doing so helps keep our air, water, and soil healthier and cleaner. Local food is more sustainable, since it costs less to be transported from a nearby farm to a local store than to be transported on a truck across the country or on a boat from across the world. At grocery stores, food typically comes labeled with its origin, allowing you to choose the foods that arrive from the closest geographical location.

Also important to note is that even though some smaller local farmers cannot afford the USDA Organic certification, you're likely to learn when you talk to them that their foods are of high quality, and they tend to use organic, sustainable, and humane farming practices.

For your baby, fresh organic foods are usually preferred over canned or frozen when it comes to flavor. Fresh food is just that—fresh-tasting! But frozen organic foods have perks, too. Often, frozen organic vegetables or fruit offer a good alternative to fresh produce because they are picked at peak ripeness and frozen, rather than sitting at the store. They, too, can be rich in flavor and nutrients. Frozen fruit and vegetables can last a long time in the freezer, and are quick to heat up on the stove. However, avoid steaming food in the bags they come in. Heating plastic in the microwave leaks plastic into the food it's surrounding, which increases chemical exposure and associated health risks. When necessary, choose organic canned goods as long as they are BPA-free (more on BPA on page 39).

Food Labeling

Organic foods are grown with methods that follow organic farming guide-lines. Produce that is labeled USDA Organic meets strict criteria in many areas, including soil quality, weed and pest control, and additives, and the produce is cultivated using natural products and specific farming methods. Meat that is certified USDA Organic comes from animals raised in conditions that are conducive to natural behaviors, fed 100 percent organic food, and not given antibiotics or hormones. Organic foods are free of toxins that can come in the form of pesticides on conventional (non-organic) foods, artifi-cial dyes, added colors or preservatives, industrial waste, or even fluoride in poultry from animal feed.

The following definitions can help you decipher labels and choose the best food when shopping for your baby. If you're unable to find a label on pro-duce that says "organic," you can simply look on its PLU sticker. A PLU code is a five-digit number. A PLU that begins with "9" means organic produce. A PLU that begins with a 3 or 4 usually means conventional produce. Produce from local farmers may not have a PLU code.

ORGANIC LABELING

100% USDA Organic: 100 percent certified organic processing, no GMOs.

USDA Organic: 95 percent or greater of certified organic ingredients, no GMOs.

Made with organic ingredients: Food with this label must contain at least 70 percent certified organic ingredients and may contain up to 30 percent non-organic ingredients. However, all ingredients must be produced with-out GMOs.

OTHER LABELS

All-natural: This label may be one of the most misleading labels of all. There is no official definition for this term by the FDA, but generally the FDA considers the term to mean free of artificial ingredients and preservatives, including artificial colors. "All-natural" does not indicate whether the food is of nutritional benefit and it does not address whether the food was produced with pesticides or other processing methods.

Antibiotic-free/Hormone-free: Free from the use of antibiotics and/or hormones. This is usually a private label the manufacturer affixes.

Animal welfare approved: Animals are pasture-raised or free-range and animals are raised by independent farmers (no mass farming).

Cage-free: A cage-free label is the next best, but there isn't a guarantee how the animals were raised, meaning they still could have been in a stressful, crowded environment.

Certified humane raised and handled: The chickens have space to roam outdoors with access to a covered barn. They are also rotated, so they have access to fresh food in the grass.

Conventionally grown/raised: This is not a label as much as a category encompassing all the foods that don't have organic labels. This food may be grown with synthetic or chemical fertilizers, weeds may be controlled with chemical herbicides, and pests may be controlled with synthetic pesticides. Animals may be given growth hormones to grow bigger and faster, the food they are given is often GMO feed and non-organic. Antibiotics and medications are typically used to treat livestock, and they may or may not have access to outdoor roaming.

Free-range: This indicates the birds lived in an environment free from pesticides, hormones, and antibiotics, and were allowed to roam freely outside.

Non-GMO: The "Non-GMO Project Verified" label comes from the Non-GMO Project, an organization that has been verifying products since 2010. These products don't contain GMOs (genetically modified organisms). The organization works with more than 14,000 companies to verify non-GMO products. The GMO Project even has an app you can use at the store to scan products and determine if they're non-GMO. Note: Although many products are labeled "Non-GMO," they are not certified unless they contain the "Non-GMO Project Verified" label.

Farm-raised: The fish was raised in a tank or enclosure within a body of water, rather than in its natural habitat.

Wild-caught: The fish was caught in its natural habitat using nets, hand-lines, divers, or traps.

First-Time Parent Advice
NO MORE GUILT!

While we as parents want to offer our babies the very best foods, it's important to acknowledge that we may not meet this standard every single time. Treat yourself with kindness and compassion. Organic and homemade food is certainly a standard to strive for, but there will be busy days or budget-conscious times when store-bought food is the only option, and that's okay! You're doing the best you can for your baby simply by setting an intention for a healthful foundation.

Organic Baby Food on a Budget

As excited as I am about organic, local, sustainable food, the reality is this: I'm a mom who's conscious of our family's budget, like you. Buying organic food often comes with a more expensive price tag than conventional foods. When you can, choose organic. When you can't, offer whole and fresh foods. That's the most important thing, whether organic or conventional. It's always better to offer whole non-organic foods than no whole foods at all. Here are some additional ways to stretch your organic dollar:

Eat with the seasons. Organic in-season produce will be less expensive than off-season produce. Have you noticed the difference between buying blueberries in the summer versus in the winter? For example, you can buy organic blueberries for about $2 per pint in June, as opposed to $6 per pint in December. Fruits and vegetables taste much better when you eat them in season. The nutrient levels also are at their peak.

Choose higher impact organics. Not sure what foods to buy organic? Visit Environmental Working Group and consult their annual lists, called the Dirty Dozen and Clean Fifteen, which name the produce that is most and least affected by pesticides, respectively (page 12).

Make your own organic baby food. Making organic baby food at home is actually more cost-effective in the long run than buying store-bought baby food. If you cook in bulk, you can make 16 servings of purée and freeze them. In fact, this method makes the beginning months of feeding easier, especially if you have to travel or leave your baby with a sitter. If you prep in the evenings and make a batch over a weekend, you can plan a couple weeks' worth of food for your baby.

THE DIRTY DOZEN™ AND CLEAN FIFTEEN™

Environmental Working Group (EWG) releases a yearly shopping guide to helps direct consumers' purchases of produce. EWG's Dirty Dozen is a list of the produce with the highest amounts of pesticide residue, and the Clean Fifteen list shows those with the lowest amount of pesticide residue. Whenever possible, choose organic if the food is on the Dirty Dozen list. When your budget dictates buying non-organic produce, shop from the Clean Fifteen list.

2020 Dirty Dozen

The following produce is the most important to buy organically in 2020:

1. Strawberries
2. Spinach
3. Kale
4. Nectarines
5. Apples
6. Grapes
7. Peaches
8. Cherries
9. Pears
10. Tomatoes
11. Celery
12. Potatoes
+ Hot peppers*

2020 Clean Fifteen

The following produce is the least critical to buy organically in 2020:

1. Avocado
2. Sweet corn
3. Pineapple
4. Onions
5. Papaya
6. Sweet peas (frozen)
7. Eggplant
8. Asparagus
9. Cauliflower
10. Cantaloupe
11. Broccoli
12. Mushrooms
13. Cabbage
14. Honeydew
15. Kiwi

*According to their standard criteria, EWG does not rank peppers among the Dirty Dozen. However, since they test positive for pesticides known to be toxic to the brain (acephate, chlorpyrifos, and oxamyl), EWG has included them in their Dirty Dozen Plus™ list.

Buying Organic

Plenty of grocery stores offer organic foods, but your local farmer's market will likely be the most helpful place for finding high-quality, nutrient-rich organic foods. If you have a local CSA (community-supported agriculture), signing up for a seasonal subscription is another way to access local and in-season food.

Here are some guidelines to help you decide what organic food to buy for your baby:

FRUITS, VEGGIES, AND HERBS

It's best to consume fruits and vegetables that are fresh, local, and in season. Some commonly found spring produce are greens (lettuce, spinach, etc.), strawberries, and asparagus. Popular summer seasonal foods include zucchini squash, yellow summer squash, melons, tomatoes, cucumbers, and blackberries. Fall foods you can easily find include pears, pumpkins, winter squash, and apples. Winter selections are smaller at some farmer's markets, but seasonal items at grocery stores include sweet potatoes, citrus, dark leafy greens, and cabbage.

Berries and greens should not be bought unless you plan to use them within three to seven days, respectively. Potatoes and winter squash can be bought further in advance (even several weeks) if stored properly in a cool and dry place. Potatoes do well in dark places, to avoid turning green. Herbs can be consumed dried or fresh, and used interchangeably in most recipes. Fresh herbs keep well in a glass of water in the refrigerator, except for basil, which keeps best in water on the counter at room temperature.

When you want to buy something out of season, opt for a frozen version. Frozen foods are usually picked at peak ripeness and flash-frozen, meaning they retain more nutrient value and flavor. Organic frozen produce can be such a time-saver, as it cuts down on prep time.

Some foods keep best at room temperature, while others stay longer refrigerated. Keep these storage tips in mind:

1. *Store at room temperature:* bananas, citrus fruits, mangos, melons, pineapples, peppers, potatoes, winter squashes, tomatoes, basil (in water)
2. *Refrigerate:* apples, apricots, berries, grapes, mushrooms, summer squash, lettuce, spinach, green beans, broccoli, cauliflower, carrots, celery, cabbage, asparagus, beets, cut fruit and vegetables
3. *Move to the refrigerator when ripe:* avocado, kiwi, nectarines, peaches, plums

GRAINS, BEANS, AND LEGUMES

Your best choice is dried versions of organic grains, beans, and legumes. Second-best would be dried non-GMO. Dried varieties tend to keep well in a cool, dry place for many weeks or months. I like to store them in glass jars in the pantry or on a kitchen shelf, so I can see what's inside. Canned beans are a good occasional substitute; just make sure to look for BPA-free and organic cans. We'll delve into grains, beans, and legumes for baby, how to properly prepare them, and when to introduce them on page 36.

MEAT AND POULTRY

Meat labels to look for are grass-fed and organic, though you may not always find both on a single package. USDA Organic beef means the animal was raised without the use of any antibiotics or hormones and fed organic, non-GMO feed. Cows that are grass-fed are able to feed freely on fresh grass, and aren't fed things to increase their size as are conventionally raised cows. Grass-fed cows get a higher amount of omega-3s in their diet from the grass, increasing your antioxidant levels when you consume the meat.

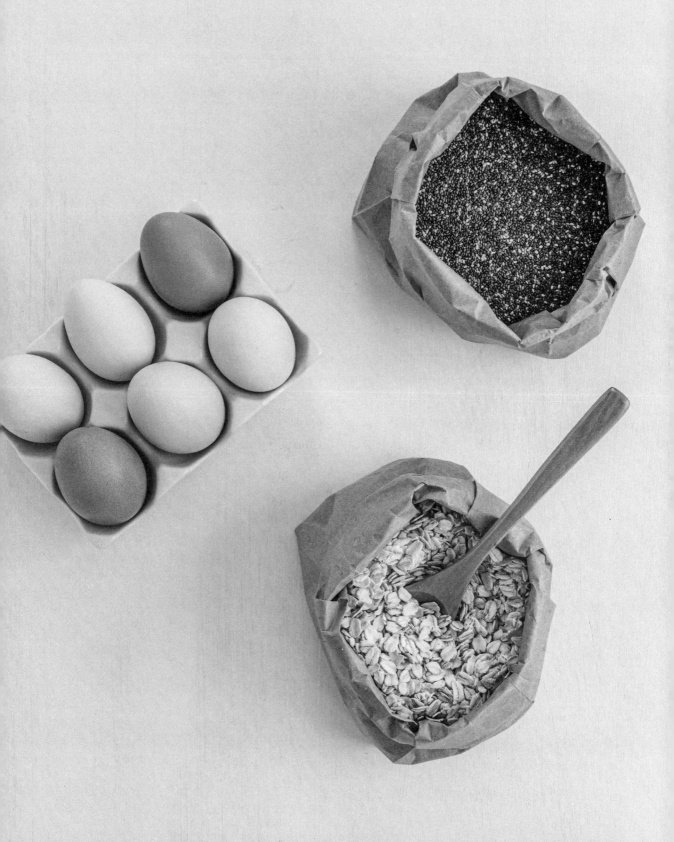

Poultry labels to look for are free-range and organic. On eggs, look for the labels organic and pasture-raised. Cage-free is next best. Quality meat, poultry, and eggs are usually found at farmer's markets, and sometimes at local CSA organizations. Buy meat and chicken fresh and freeze it if you don't plan to cook it by the "use by" date.

FISH AND SEAFOOD

If you're able to buy fish locally and fresh (considering you live near water), do it! If you can't, look for the "wild-caught" label on fresh or frozen seafood. Mercury content matters for little ones, because at high levels it can be toxic. High-mercury fish to avoid are tuna, king mackerel, swordfish, and shark. One way to remember some low-mercury (and high omega-3) fish is by the acronym SMASH: salmon, Atlantic mackerel, anchovies, sardines, and herring. Other low-mercury fish include shrimp, scallops, cod, haddock, trout, and sole. See Resources (page 234) for the link to a chart showing the mercury content of different fish.

OIL AND ANIMAL FAT

Babies need healthy sources of saturated fat and good cholesterol in the form of animal fat like grass fed-butter, and in the form of oil like olive, coconut, and avocado. For coconut and olive oils, get cold-pressed and organic if possible. Avoid oils like canola, corn, sunflower, safflower, "vegetable," peanut, cottonseed, and grapeseed. (For more on Fat and Cholesterol, see page 29.)

LET'S TALK ABOUT SUGAR

Sugar is added to almost everything nowadays. The problem is that sugar can be addictive and it also feeds yeast. Overgrowth of yeast can lead to a slew of problems for anyone, especially a baby starting solids. There is no benefit to adding refined sugar to your baby's food—babies do well with what they're given. If you give them sugar, their body will want more. Kids with high-sugar diets in childhood are more likely to battle issues with blood sugar regulation, tooth decay, and inflammation in the body. Small amounts of natural sweeteners are fine once your baby is a year old. Stick to small amounts of non-centrifugal sugar (such as rapadura, which retains some nutrients), coconut or palm sugar, blackstrap molasses (rich in vitamin B6, potassium, magnesium, and manganese), maple syrup, dates, and honey (honey is especially important to delay introducing until after age 1, as it may contain bacteria harmful to a baby. Once honey is introduced, raw and local varieties are preferable). A few of the 8- to 12-months-old recipes in this book call for a tiny amount of maple syrup, like mixed into homemade yogurt, which is safe in such a small amount.

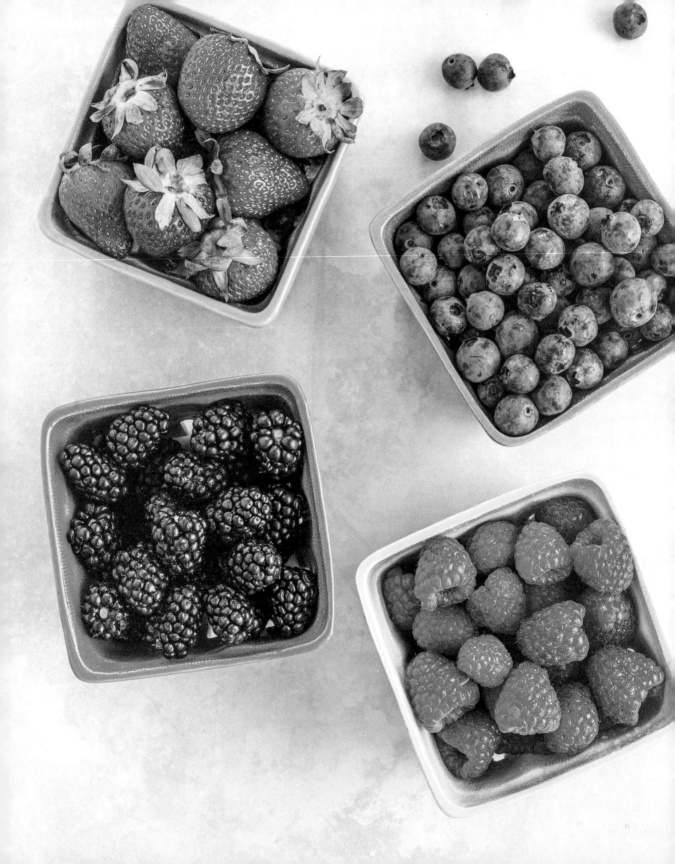

Two

Feeding & Nutrition

Preparing for your baby's first bites can be as simple as you want it to be. We'll cover some of the biggest issues regarding food introduction, including when to start solids, the two main types of feeding approaches, what critical nutrients your baby needs more of in the first year, common food allergies and intolerances, and how gagging and choking are different. Even with all of this, we'll explore how feeding should be fun!

When to Start?

As a nurse and health coach, I've seen how overwhelming it is for first-time parents to figure out when to start their baby on solids. The truth is your baby will tell you by showing feeding readiness signs. There isn't a one-size-fits-all approach to feeding a little one. Instead, the following guidelines will help you know what to watch for in your baby so you can give them solids at their perfect time. Not the time Grandma wants, the month your pediatrician says, or when your best friend gave her baby solids.

There is no rush when starting solids, as fun as it may be, because these first foods will have a big impact on the immune system. Rushing now can result in future challenges. The majority of experts recommend nothing outside of mom's breast milk or formula for the first 6 months of life. The World Health Organization (WHO) and American Academy of Pediatrics (AAP) strongly recommend not introducing anything else before 4 months, and that you wait until as close to 6 months as possible. Before 6 months, babies do not make all the necessary enzymes to digest food, have underdeveloped kidneys, lack favorable bacteria for digestion, and have an open/leaky gut (see page 45). So when solids are introduced too early, it increases their risk of food intolerances and allergies.

Once your baby meets the following six readiness signs, they are generally giving you the thumbs-up that they are ready to go. Let these be the gold standard for intuitively following your baby's lead, and introducing foods at the right time. Note that some babies show these signs at 5 ½ months, others at 8 months. All babies meet these signs at different stages, just like any other milestone.

1. *Sits unsupported, or with minimal assistance.* This is important because the digestive system is muscular. When baby's abdominal muscles are strong enough to support the core, it's indicative that the digestive muscles are capable of digesting food.

2. *Indicates they are done feeding by turning head from breast/bottle.* This ability allows the baby to communicate when they are full or if their body is saying "no" to whatever we are feeding them (for example, if they have a tummy ache). Tuning in and respecting these cues are important because, often, the first sign of an illness is a change in your baby's appetite.

3. *Opens mouth when something comes toward face/mouth.* Babies' oral exploration is key in their development. They taste and feel new textures by doing this.

4. *Can close lips around spoon.* This motor skill shows readiness to accept food into their mouth.

5. *Shows interest by watching others.* Sometimes this happens around 4 months, which gives parents mixed signals that maybe they are ready to eat. But at this age (and for the next several months), they will put almost anything in their mouth, including dirt!

6. *Loses the tongue thrust instinct.* This is an involuntary reflex when babies push food or other objects out of their mouth. Its primary purpose is to prevent them from choking or aspirating, and to help them get a good latch when nursing or feeding. It usually goes away around the time baby is ready to start solids, as baby learns how to chew and swallow.

What to Expect, Stage by Stage

In this book, we'll explore very first bites of food, working up to purées, ensuring variability in textures and flavors, and incorporating your own family meals into bite-size meals for your baby as they grow into toddlerhood and early childhood. The goal is not to have you making something totally different for your baby all the time, but instead working toward offering your child "big-people" food with the rest of the family.

The recipes are organized by first foods (bone broth and avocado), purées (fruits, vegetables, meats, and seafood), mixing and matching foods, finger foods and chunky mashes, and toddler and family meals, as well as must-have snacks for your busy toddler. You'll also find Superfoods for Baby (page 49) if you want to take nutrition up a notch. As your baby progresses through each stage, follow your baby's lead, as the following are just guidelines. Each child will be different, and when they are going through a growth spurt or feeling ill, the portions and stages will vary.

6 TO 8 MONTHS

The concept of baby food between 6 to 8 months is more about introducing the idea of foods. It's more important for them to get the taste and experience than to "get the serving in." The primary source of nutrition is still breast milk or formula. At this age, you'll introduce the rhythm of eating alongside their current daily patterns. The only big focus here is on offering iron-rich foods.

Time of day: After offering your baby breast milk or formula in the morning, you can offer a mid-morning solid food. Morning is best so you can monitor for any adverse reactions throughout the day.

Amount: 2 to 4 tablespoons of food, give or take (less to start). Follow your baby's lead here and use your discretion. When they start losing interest, they're done.

Texture: You can offer puréed-texture foods or some sliced soft-cooked foods. If you offer a purée, the consistency should be thin and watery, just a little thicker than formula or breast milk. If they enjoy and master that, you can make it a bit lumpier.

8 TO 12 MONTHS

Around 8 to 9 months, you will start to establish more of a pattern of feeding, rather than random tastings. You'll still want to avoid any strict schedule.

Time of day: A sample pattern would be: wake up, nurse/bottle, mid-morning meal, nurse/bottle before an afternoon nap, dinner meal with the family, and nurse/bottle before bed.

Amount: 2 tablespoons to ½ cup per meal, following baby's lead

Texture: Variety in texture and flavor is desired here, foods should be thicker than they have been so far, and can include some very soft, mushy lumps (easily mashable with their hard gums, even if they have no teeth).

12 TO 18 MONTHS

At 12 months, breastfeeding for toddlers varies from child to child. Some toddlers nurse one to four times in a 24-hour period, and that is totally normal alongside solid food. Formula-fed babies often take a bottle or cup in the morning and in the evening. Some toddlers at 12 to 18 months slowly transition away from formula and begin on another form of dairy, such as goat's, cow's, or other alternatives (see page 163).

Time of day: About three meals and two to three snacks a day

Amount: ¼ cup to 1 cup of food per meal, following baby's lead

Texture: Children are mostly eating foods with "big-people" textures, with caution and safety adjustments (mashing, cutting, cooking, etc.) to choking hazards (such as berries, soft breads, cherry tomatoes, nuts, grapes, chunks of food, popcorn, and raw vegetables).

Hybrid Baby-Led Feeding Approach

Before high-speed blenders became a regular kitchen appliance, what did we do? Moms offered mashed cooked vegetables, pre-chewed meats (really!), or simply sized and sliced whole foods in "baby-led feeding" fashion.

While this book covers a lot of beginning purées and mashes that you can offer your baby with a spoon, there are finger food recipes, too, that align more with baby-led feeding, also known as baby-led weaning, or BLW. This method allows the baby to be in charge of feeding themselves (see Resources, page 234 for more information on baby-led feeding). You can also incorporate baby-led feeding into your spoon-feeding plan for a hybrid approach. Some of the benefits of baby-led feeding are that it:

- Gives your baby control over what and how much they eat, thereby promoting a healthy relationship with food
- Supports fine motor development and chewing skills
- Helps establish your baby's intuitive eating sense (knowing when they are full, and when to stop) which reduces the risk of obesity, according to research

However, baby-led feeding does come with down sides, including increased food waste, messy feedings, and potential gagging or choking, which can be scary for you and your baby.

If you'd like to try to incorporate baby-led feeding, remember that it's up to you and your baby and that you can change things around if it's not working for either of you. Do whatever you feel the most at ease with.

FINGER-SAFE FOODS

If you plan to do a hybrid feeding approach with baby-led weaning, foods will need to be cut in a specific shape (length and thickness).

AGES 6 TO 8 MONTHS: A general rule of thumb for this age is soft finger foods, cut into long strips that are about your finger length and width. Try sliced avocado or banana in this fashion and make sure they aren't overripe or mushy, so baby can grip the slices.

AGES 9 TO 12 MONTHS: Around this age, smaller bite-size pieces of food are appropriate for babies to practice their pincer grasp. Try soft-cooked vegetables (like roasted beets or roasted sweet potatoes in strips), soft-cooked meats, very ripe pieces of fruit (like mango or peach), or smashed blueberries. For any round foods like cherry tomatoes or grapes, you'll want to quarter them and not halve them, to minimize choking risk.

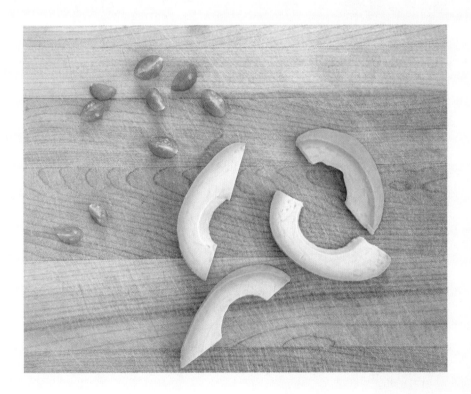

Baby's Nutrition

Babies need a lot of nutrients, especially in the first year of life as their brain and body are rapidly developing. If baby is breastfed, a healthful mom's diet provides most of these nutrients, but once they start eating foods, babies need an extra food source to boost some of these micronutrients if they are consuming less breast milk. Iron is the greatest need in the 6- to 9-month age range (see page 27 for more on iron needs).

The recipes in this book can help ensure that your baby gets adequate daily amounts of the necessary nutrients, but it's important to know they may not meet this standard every single day. In the early stages, your baby will still be obtaining most of their nutrition and calories from either breast milk or formula.

If you are thinking about raising a plant-based child, it's important to work with a certified nutritionist and make your pediatrician aware of your decision. While there is certainly reason to be conscious of overconsuming commercialized, poor-quality, factory-farmed meats, there are also risks with omitting animal foods altogether in a baby's diet, and a good plant-based diet will require being well-informed on the subject. While the essential nutrients a baby needs are extremely easy to obtain from an animal source, they can be more difficult to get through a plant-based diet. It's not impossible, but usually requires supplementation of a few nutrients; in particular, vitamins B_{12} and D_3.

VITAMIN D_3

Vitamin D_3 is essential for baby's immunity, gut health, and healthy sleep cycles, and aids in the absorption of calcium and phosphorus for strong bones. Vitamin D_3 is the type of vitamin D our bodies make from natural sunlight. Since babies aren't supposed to be in the sun for long amounts of time, the AAP recommends a supplement of 400 IU daily for infants.

Primary sources: 20 minutes of sun exposure daily, oily fish (mackerel, salmon), egg yolk, cheese, and liver

Supplementation: If you are nursing and taking a daily vitamin D supplement of 5,000 IU or greater, your baby may not need a supplement. Otherwise, babies under 12 months need 400 IU of vitamin D daily, as recommended by the AAP. Formula usually has this added. Babies on a plant-based diet will need supplementation.

IRON

Iron is literal brain food. It supports the normal protection of the nervous system and brain cells. Since iron stores start depleting around 6 months, it is essential that babies get a boost through solid food. Iron-deficiency damage can be irreversible. Babies between 6 and 12 months old need the same levels of iron as an adult man (11mg), and then 7mg thereafter from ages 1 to 3 years.

Babies can get dietary iron in two ways: heme iron sources and non-heme iron sources. Heme iron is the most absorbable type of iron, and is only found in animal sources. Non-heme iron is a much less absorbable type of iron, and can be found in plant-based sources like leafy greens, beans, and nuts. For plant-based iron sources, it helps to pair the food with foods that are high in vitamin C to enhance absorption and usability, and soak them to reduce phytic acid, which blocks absorption.

Heme sources: Red meat, liver, marrow, poultry, lamb, fish, egg yolks

Non-heme sources: Lentils and beans, dried apricots, leafy greens, nuts, seeds, chickpeas, spirulina

Supplementation: For plant-based babies, talk with your pediatrician or nutritionist to discuss your baby's individual needs.

CALCIUM

Calcium is essential for bone and teeth development, blood clotting, muscle function, a regular heart rhythm, and hormone and nervous system regulation. Adequate calcium levels are critical for babies, and really for all of us! A baby's calcium needs are 260mg daily for ages 6 to 12 months and 700mg daily for ages 1 to 3 years.

Food sources: Salmon, leafy greens, almond butter, cheese, beans, broccoli, and fermented foods

Supplementation: For plant-based babies, talk with your pediatrician or nutritionist to discuss your baby's individual needs.

PROBIOTICS

Probiotics are essential for diversifying good gut bacteria, which equates to a healthy immune and digestive system (regular bowel movements, etc.). Many infant probiotics carry similar strains that support the digestive system with a purpose for each strain. It is really important to provide babies with a probiotic supplement, especially in the following three situations:

1. Baby was born via C-section.
2. Baby takes formula.
3. Baby has had antibiotics.

Through the birth canal and through breast milk, babies receive specific strains of probiotics to help colonize their digestive system, and thus their immune system, since the two go hand in hand. If your baby needed an antibiotic, the antibiotic did what it was supposed to by wiping out all the bad bacteria, but it also wiped out the good bacteria. It can take up to 2 years for that gut to rebuild the good bacteria, so supplementing with a probiotic can help reshape it!

Food sources: Plain yogurt, kefir, and fermented foods such as kimchi, sauerkraut brine, sauerkraut, and sourdough bread

Supplementation: Supplement if your baby was born via C-section; if antibiotics were given during pregnancy, labor, or directly to baby since birth; or if the mother has a history of yeast infections.

OMEGA-3S AND DHA/EPA

Omega-3s are responsible for keeping the blood thin and protecting the nervous system, while helping your baby's growth and development. Two important types of omega-3 fatty acids your baby needs are DHA and EPA, which are usually found together.

Food sources for omega-3s: Cold-water fish like salmon and sardines, chia, flax meal, and walnuts

Supplementation: Choose cod liver oil supplements, which contain adequate DHA and omegas (and are also rich in vitamins A and D). DHA supplements (sometimes with DHA sourced from marine algae) are available that can cater to plant-based babies.

FAT AND CHOLESTEROL

Although fat and cholesterol have been demonized in the past, offering a high-fat diet to your baby is absolutely vital. A few biological things to know about babies and fats/cholesterol:

Breast milk is comprised of over 50 percent fat. About half is saturated fat along with a liberal amount of cholesterol. No wonder we need to continue to offer these good fats to baby once they begin nursing less! Fats are also needed to absorb fat-soluble vitamins (A, D, E, and K) and to fuel the nervous system and brain to function properly.

About 60 percent of the brain is made of fat! In order for your baby's brain to keep growing at a rapid speed, fat is essential. Saturated fats make up every cell wall in your baby's body, supporting the heart, lungs, bones, brain, and nervous tissue.

Cholesterol enables the body to function in many ways. It supports a healthy digestive system by strengthening the intestinal lining. It's also needed for healthy hormone production and for vitamin D metabolism.

Food sources: Avocado, coconut oil, avocado oil, nut butters, and full-fat dairy such as butter, yogurt, and cheese

Supplementation: For plant-based babies, talk with your pediatrician or nutritionist to discuss your baby's individual needs.

TAKING CARE OF YOU

While taking care of baby is of primary importance, we can't forget about ourselves! As parents, we need to keep our diets well-rounded and get sunshine, fresh air, and hydration to help optimize our immune system, and offer our bodies the nutrients it needs. To stay healthy, make sure you:

- Eat a diet rich in organic whole foods and fresh vegetables and fruits.
- Rotate between oily fish, meats, and poultry.
- Incorporate healthy fats like coconut oil, avocado, nuts, and animals fats such as grass-fed butter.
- Try recipes that fuel up the entire family such as Nut Butter Power Bites (page 192), Banana Mini Muffins (page 149), and Soaked Granola (page 189).

Breastfeeding Mothers

Breastfeeding mothers should continue taking prenatal vitamins with folate and methylcobalamin, also known as 5-MTHF. However, this is not a replacement for a nutrient-rich diet. Also, a low-carb diet is not ideal if you are nursing. Here are some additional dietary recommendations:

TAKE AN OMEGA-3 SUPPLEMENT LIKE COD LIVER OIL. Adequate fat in your diet is good for brain health and combats "mommy brain."

STAY HYDRATED. Each time you sit down to nurse, grab a glass of water. If you take your weight and divide it by two, you'll get the number of ounces of water you need daily to operate at an optimal level.

GET CREATIVE WITH HYDRATION. Warm teas and bone broths are also great for nursing mothers, and they count toward hydration. Caffeinated drinks do not.

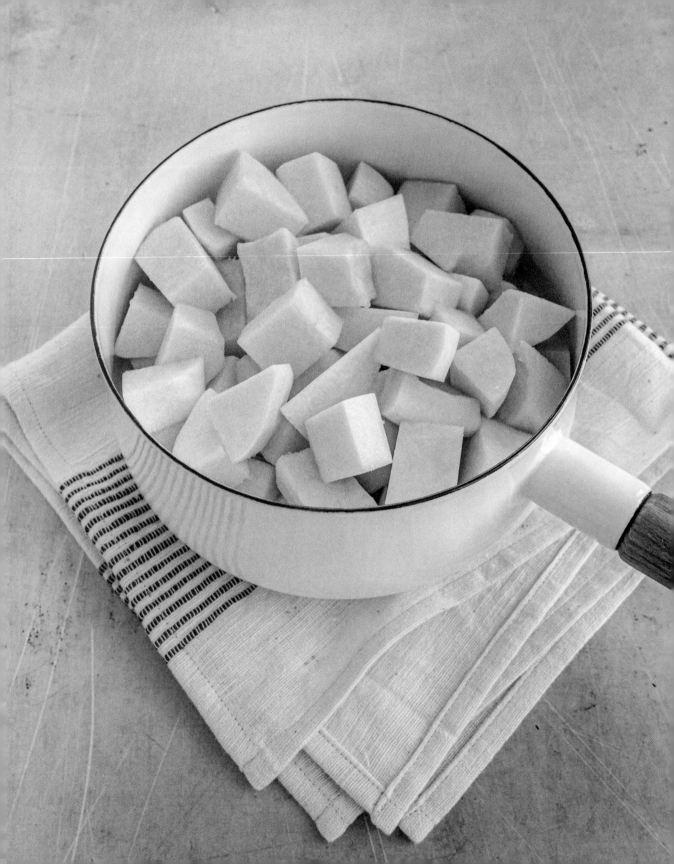

Three
Cooking for Baby

One of my favorite things about homemade baby food is how simple it is to make! In the early stages of feeding solids, you'll cook the food until it's soft, then either mash it or purée it. It's all about offering nutritious foods you are probably already eating, but in a safe way. In this chapter, we'll go over preparation, cooking, and storage of your baby's food, as well as feeding gear such as high chairs and sippy cups.

Food Safety

All the basics of food safety apply to baby food as well. You probably already know these tips and rules, but it's always good to have a refresher and reassure yourself that you're doing everything you can to keep food prep clean and healthy:

Clean your hands and your tools. Wash your hands with soap and warm water before you begin. Wash any tools, including knives, and clean the countertop where you are preparing food.

Wash your hands throughout. When you switch between cutting raw meat or handling raw eggs to slicing veggies, rewash hands (and knives) to avoid cross-contamination.

Thaw food in the refrigerator overnight. This allows for safe, slow thawing. You can thaw individual frozen food cubes in a bowl in the refrigerator overnight, then reheat them on the stove or in a bowl of hot water.

Pay attention to perishables. Don't leave perishable foods out on the counter for more than 2 hours.

Store food safely. In general, most cooked foods are good in the refrigerator for up to 3 to 4 days and up to 3 months in the freezer.

Fruit and Vegetable Prep

Washing produce before use is important, particularly if you are buying conventional food. Pesticides, bacteria, and dirt can linger on the leaves and skins of foods. Keep in mind that bacteria can also linger on organic produce from transit to the store and people touching them while shopping.

A good way to wash produce is by giving it a vinegar and water soak when you get home before putting it away, as vinegar can clean bacteria, fungi, and pesticides off produce. To do this, simply fill a clean sink or a large bowl with lukewarm water and white vinegar in a 3:1 ratio. Submerge the produce, including the ones with hard outer rinds (such as oranges and lemons), for about 10 minutes, rinse with clean water, dry, and store. However, avoid soaking potatoes, mushrooms, or berries. You can quickly dunk berries in the vinegar/water bath for a minute or so, but they can get soggy if not dried well. Larger produce like melons and squash can also be dunked in the vinegar/water bath, but I prefer to spray them with the same ratio of vinegar and water in a spray bottle and then wipe it off.

When you're ready to prepare the fruits or vegetables for cooking, clean the countertops with a gentle but effective disinfectant like vinegar and water. (You can fill a spray bottle with a 1:1 mix of water and vinegar.) Make sure to use a cutting board dedicated for produce. If cooking the produce, be sure to cut foods in relatively similar sizes so that they cook at the same speed.

Meat, Poultry, and Seafood Prep

Before cutting beef, poultry, or seafood, clean the countertops with your 1:1 vinegar and water solution. Use hot water and soap to wash your knife and cutting board, washing in between if you are switching between any meat, poultry, or seafood. To thaw any of these from frozen, place the meat in a large enough bowl in the refrigerator overnight. Meat does not require rinsing prior to preparation, as the bacteria will be destroyed by cooking. Just make sure to keep these raw ingredients separate from other foods, particularly fresh produce.

Grains, Beans, and Legumes Prep

Grains, beans, and legumes have one thing in common: they contain phytic acid, or an "antinutrient." This does not make them bad foods; just harder for our body to digest, which sometimes results in inflammation or bloating. Phytic acid helps keep the food from germinating and spoiling before it's time to prepare and eat. Think of phytic acid as a shield. Another issue is that when left alone, phytic acid can bind with important minerals and vitamins and block their absorption. Calcium, magnesium, copper, iron, and especially zinc are bound by phytic acid, preventing the intestinal tract from absorbing them—unless they are broken down first.

When we introduce grains, beans, or legumes to babies, they should be properly prepared. Soaking enhances digestion, makes nutrients absorbable, and reduces cook time. Large amounts of partially or undigested grains, beans, or legumes can make it difficult for the body to break down the complex starches. By properly preparing these foods through soaking, the body can more easily digest and absorb the nutrients from them. It's really quite easy to soak them; it just requires a little bit of forethought. Once you get used to it, it'll become a habit!

HOW TO SOAK

1. Use a clean glass, ceramic, or stainless-steel bowl. Make sure to use a non-reactive bowl, since the acid may react with cast iron, plastic, copper, or aluminum.
2. Add the desired amount of grains, beans, or legumes. Cover the food you're soaking with at least 1 inch of warm, filtered water.
3. Add 1 to 2 teaspoons of acid (cider vinegar, lemon juice, or whey) per cup of dried grain, bean, or legume.
4. Let soak according to the following soak time list (see page 37).
5. Discard the water after soaking and rinse food well.

If you only have an hour before cooking or forgot to soak them, it's okay. Even an hour of soaking with an acid can break down some of the phytic acid. The following soak times are for raw beans, but soaking canned beans even for an hour is beneficial and can unlock a broader nutrient profile.

- **Adzuki beans:** 8 to 12 hours
- **Almonds:** 8 to 12 hours
- **Black beans:** 8 to 12 hours
- **Cashews:** 6 hours maximum
- **Chickpeas:** 12 hours
- **Hazelnuts:** 8 to 12 hours
- **Lentils:** 7 hours
- **Macadamia nuts:** 2 hours maximum
- **Millet or quinoa:** 5 hours
- **Oats:** 6 hours minimum
- **Pecans:** 6 hours
- **Pistachios:** 8 hours
- **Pumpkin seeds:** 8 hours
- **Rice (preferably black, wild, or brown):** 7 hours minimum
- **Walnuts:** 4 hours

Cooking Essentials

Aim to stock your kitchen with quality, non-toxic cookware, and utensils made of stainless steel, cast iron, wood, or toxic-free ceramic. It is best to avoid the use of plastic, especially in the kitchen (see BPA and Other Toxins, page 39). The following is a list of the cookware to have on hand to make the recipes in this book:

Prep Tools

- Wood cutting boards
- Chef's knife
- Paring knife
- Vegetable peeler

Cooking Equipment

- Medium stainless-steel saucepan with lid
- Large stainless-steel stockpot (about 6 quarts) with lid
- Steamer basket
- Rimmed baking sheet
- Mini muffin pan
- High-speed blender or immersion blender

Freezing and Storage

- Silicone ice cube trays
- Silicone zip-top freezer bags or airtight glass containers
- Small glass jars (can be old glass condiment containers)
- Quart or half-gallon Mason jars

Feeding Essentials

Spoons, bibs, and high chairs—oh my! The options are countless, but it's best to keep baby feeding equipment simple, using a few quality pieces that can grow with your child and last for future children. See Resources (page 234) for my brand and product recommendations.

BIBS

Most bibs do a good job at keeping little ones clean, but consider ones made of silicone that wipe clean and have a food catcher at the bottom, or smock-style bibs, which keep arms clean and are easy to throw in the washer.

TABLEWARE

In all of your tableware, avoid plastic, as it contains more toxins. Look for silicone spoons or forks for early eaters. You can advance to easy-grip stainless-steel forks and spoons once baby is closer to 12 months. The main things to look for are simple designs, a good gripping piece for little hands, and quality materials.

For bowls, silicone works really well; there are also suction cup bowls that can thwart your little one from dumping their food. Silicone tableware is also sturdy, dishwasher-safe, naturally bacteria-resistant, stain-resistant, and even oven-safe in some cases.

Sippy cups are one of the things I see pile up in parents' cabinets. Look for stainless-steel ones with an ergonomic design that teach your child to sip from an open cup, as well as designs that prevent food from getting trapped. Another good feature is spill-proof for those times when they get dumped upside-down.

HIGH CHAIRS

Some things to consider when choosing high chairs are space (folding vs. non-folding), safety, and ease of cleaning. I recommend choosing one that fits your space and budget, with one key feature to look for: a footrest. This helps with safety, comfort, and ease of eating. The footrest gives babies something to push against when they gag, allowing them to utilize their abdominal muscles.

BPA AND OTHER TOXINS

You may have heard about the importance of "BPA-free" products. Bisphenol A, or BPA, is a chemical found in plastic that poses great health risks. Research has shown that BPA plays a significant role in the development of endocrine disorders, including but not limited to female and male infertility, early-onset puberty, increased risks of cancers, and metabolic disorders (such as PCOS). For children, BPA exposure can cause an increase in anxiety, hyperactivity, and obesity. Because of this, it's important to stay away from using plastics in the kitchen. In addition, you'll want avoid the following toxin-containing items:

- Non-stick pans that contain Teflon, as the World Health Organization lists it as a possible carcinogen
- Aluminum, including foil—aluminum is a known neurotoxin and is found in the brains of Alzheimer's patients
- Ceramic cookware, which is often coated with a glaze that contains lead

NO-STRESS COOKING

As parents, we want to make life easier without compromising the nutrients we offer to our baby, and find more time in our busy lives for enjoyment. Here are some tips for stress-free cooking:

WASH VEGETABLES AND CHOP THEM FOR THE WEEK'S RECIPES. Do this as soon as you get home from the store. This will make it easier for quick prep when you're ready to cook.

MAKE A WEEKLY MEAL PLAN AND ROTATE IT. Vary the recipes but keep a general guide of something like this: Taco Tuesday, Leftover Wednesday, One-Pot Meal Thursday, Pasta Friday. Each week, I like to switch it up on the tacos, rotating a taco bowl, fish tacos, or chicken or beef tacos.

DO A FAMILY GROCERY TRIP! It can be fun to involve the family and have an extra set of hands from your partner. With the new practice of social distancing, maintain the guidelines in your geographical location and use your discretion for family grocery shopping trips.

MAKE IT A DATE. Ditch the previous idea altogether, get a sitter, and go on a late-night grocery excursion, baby-free! Sometimes it's therapeutic to have time to browse and not have to worry about nap schedules.

ORDER GROCERIES ONLINE. It can feel like a luxury to order food from your computer, then have someone package it up for you. Any service fees are offset by the fact that you aren't impulse buying. And you're saving time and gas, so it's a win-win.

TAKE INVENTORY BEFORE MAKING A SHOPPING LIST. Dig through your freezer, pantry, and refrigerator each week. This will keep you aware of what you've got versus what you need.

DOUBLE-BATCH RECIPES, AND FREEZE HALF FOR BUSY NIGHTS. Recipes from this book that freeze great include Coconut Chicken Curry with Carrots and Potatoes (page 142), Four-Bean Chili with Veggies (page 210), Chickpea Minestrone Soup (page 227), Lamb Meatballs with Tzatziki Dipping Sauce (page 223; make the tzatziki sauce fresh) and Blender Oat Pancakes (page 172).

EAT LEFTOVER DINNERS FOR LUNCH THE NEXT DAY. This is another benefit of double-batching recipes the day before.

START A RECIPE COLLECTION. When you find a favorite, print it to keep on hand. Whenever you're looking for inspiration, sift through your recipe collection. The more you make a dish, the easier it becomes to throw it together without thought.

SWAP WITH A FRIEND. Once a week, arrange to double-batch and share your meal with a friend or neighbor, while on another night they double-batch and share with you.

GET CREATIVE WITH BOWLS. Talk about eating the rainbow! Bowls are a meal-in-one that you can create from whatever you've got on hand—think brown rice, couscous, quinoa, greens, cheese, sauerkraut, capers, fish, meats, mushrooms, avocado—you're only limited by your imagination. Top with a squeeze of lemon, some sesame oil, or sour cream. This works well with leftover vegetables and meats. For those who don't like it all mixed together, set it up in a make-your-own-bowl bar so everyone, including toddlers, can keep the ingredients separate if they prefer it that way.

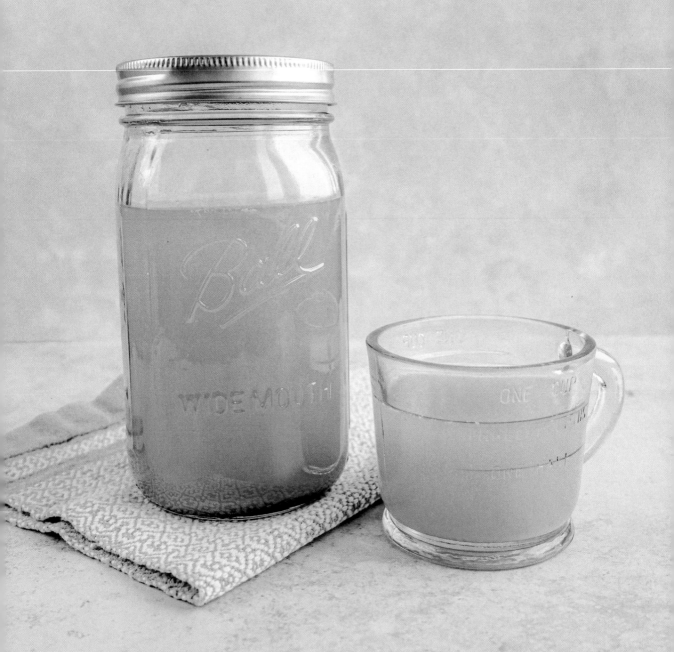

Four

Baby's First Foods

Babies are ready for their first food at different times, but you can generally expect readiness between 6 and 7 months. You can revisit the readiness list on page 21 to determine if your baby is showing signs they are developmentally able to start. Once your baby has given the green light, what exactly should you choose as their first bite? Let's explore.

Food #1: Bone Broth

I recommend starting solids with a traditional food our ancestors in many cultures have been feeding babies for hundreds of years: bone broth. For example, in traditional Chinese medicine, using the healing properties of bone broth dates back more than 2,500 years. Generations later, our grandmothers (and now you!) are still making broth. This well-known "remedy" for cold and flu treatment actually holds up scientifically. Ailments that affect connective tissue (found in the gastrointestinal tract, joints, skin, lungs, and muscles around the blood) are supported by the gelatin that cooks down from the bones, creating that rich bone broth. The bones and cartilage break down into collagen, which breaks down into gelatin. The more gelatin, the merrier. Collagen comes from the Greek word *kolla*, which means glue. And that's just what the collagen/gelatin do to the digestive tract: hold it together.

Bone broth benefits come from the gelatin that comes from cooked collagen in bones. Homemade bone broth is easy to make and best for baby because it tends to be more nutrient-dense; plus, you control the ingredients (see recipe, page 47). The quality and type of bones matter, too—knuckle bones, in particular, contain hefty amounts of collagen. The collagen in gelatin-rich broth helps seal a baby's naturally born "leaky gut" (or the small gaps in their gut's membrane lining). Here are some benefits of bone broth:

- Helps prevent food allergies or intolerances by strengthening the gut lining with its collagen and gelatin-rich components
- Builds strong bones and teeth with its absorbable magnesium and calcium
- Improves immune and digestive function with its amino acids

LEAKY GUT IN BABIES

You might be wondering, *my newborn has a leaky gut?* Yes, but it's not a bad thing! Babies are born with a leaky gut on purpose, as it allows nutrients and antibody particles from breastfeeding or formula-feeding to pass through the gut wall and into the bloodstream. As baby gets older, these gaps need to be maintained well and not be too spaced out, which can cause too many larger particles to pass through. In other words, the gaps in the leaky gut need to be sealed.

If those gaps are too big (or "leaky") when foods are introduced into baby's digestive system, these foods can pass through the permeable gut and into the bloodstream. When this happens, the body sees these whole or partially digested proteins as a foreign invader and attacks. That specific food is put into the immune system's memory as an invader, activating an allergic immune response the next time it sees it.

Each baby's genetic makeup and toxin exposures vary, which is why babies are affected by leaky gut to different degrees. The following are some common signs associated with leaky gut:

- Abdominal distention (tautness/tightness and fullness)
- Gas
- Colic
- Spitting up
- Hives
- Rashes
- Eczema
- Nasal and sinus congestion
- Swollen mouth
- Cough
- Trouble breathing

For some, the following longer-term issues may develop, including:

- Lifelong food allergies
- Autoimmune disorders
- Digestive issues
- Inflammation
- Overstimulation of the immune system
- Nutrient deficiencies
- Chronic illness
- Cognitive dysfunction

The important thing to remember is that when the leaky gut has outlived its initial usefulness as a method for dispersing nutrients into the bloodstream and food is about to be introduced, bone broth is an excellent first food to assist in the sealing of the gut (through the collagen and gelatin it provides) and help protect against any complications related to leaky gut.

WHAT ABOUT RICE CEREAL?

Until recently, rice cereal was the number-one recommendation as baby's first food, largely because it was thought to be low-allergenic and it's iron-fortified. Although babies do need a big iron boost around 6 to 9 months, rice cereal is an outdated recommendation and not the ideal choice because it's refined (essentially stripped of its natural nutrients). The specific type of iron the body needs is heme iron, available only from meat, poultry, and fish. Heme iron is the most absorbable type of iron. Iron-fortified rice cereal only contains about 4 percent absorbable iron, and unfortunately, blocks the absorption of zinc.

In addition, babies are born biologically intolerant to grains. This doesn't mean they can never have grains or that grains are bad. It just means we need to be aware of their digestive enzymes and developing digestive system when we introduce foods like grains to the gut. Babies need the digestive enzyme pancreatic amylase to break down big starches like rice cereal, but they don't actually possess larger amounts of this essential digestive enzyme until closer to 12 to 18 months. So you'll see that some of the recipes in this book, particularly for babies under a year old, use gluten-free flours such as coconut flour, almond flour, or oat flour.

Bone Broth

PREP TIME: 10 minutes, plus 1 hour to soak the bones   **COOK TIME:** 24 hours
FREEZER-FRIENDLY · **DAIRY-FREE** · **GLUTEN-FREE** · **NUT-FREE**

This vital first-food recipe is meant to be made ahead and frozen in silicone trays. To thaw, place a cube in a jar in the refrigerator overnight. You can serve bone broth warm to your baby using a spoon, small sippy cup, bottle, oral medicine syringe, or as a frozen cube in a mesh feeder. You can continue giving bone broth daily to your baby throughout the first year and alongside new foods. You can serve it alone or cook with it as your baby grows. **MAKES ABOUT 3 QUARTS**

2 to 3 pounds beef knuckle bones

12 cups filtered water

2 tablespoons apple cider vinegar

1   In a large stockpot, cover the bones with 6 cups of filtered water. Add the apple cider vinegar and let soak for 1 hour.

2   Add the remaining 6 cups of water to the pot. Bring to a gentle boil over high heat, then cover and simmer over low heat for 24 hours, or up to 72 hours. Watch the broth closely for the first 2 hours, skimming the surface to remove any foam or excess fat. Do not leave the pot unattended overnight. You can remove it from the heat, cool the broth overnight in the refrigerator, and continue simmering the next morning. (This can also be made in a slow cooker.)

3   Remove and discard the bones. Using a fine-mesh strainer, strain the broth. Use cheesecloth to do a final straining, if needed. Set aside and let cool.

4   Pour the broth into silicone trays and freeze, in batches if necessary.

Storage: Refrigerate the remaining broth in Mason jars until ready to freeze.

Tip: You can use a chicken carcass, including feet and neck (cook for 12 to 24 hours), as well as bison, lamb, or pork bones (cook for 24 hours, minimum). Also, this simple broth without vegetables is recommended when making your first batch. Vegetable scraps from any already introduced vegetables may be added once your baby has had them individually without any reaction.

FEEDING SUCCESS

As you get ready to feed your baby, you'll want to set yourself and your baby up for short- and long-term success. The following tips create a happy eating experience for your baby:

GIVE FIRST BITES OF FOOD IN THE MORNING. Babies are often in the best mood when they wake up. This also allows you to monitor for a food allergy or intolerance throughout the day.

MINIMIZE DISTRACTIONS. Turn off the television and avoid using electronic distractions to get your baby to eat. Pull up a chair in front of your baby, and spend mindful eating time with them.

SIT BABY STRAIGHT UP, NOT RECLINED. Ideally, they should be in a high chair where they can plant their feet. This also allows them to use their core muscles easily if they're gagging.

OFFER YOUR BABY A SMALL AMOUNT AT FIRST. You can put it directly on their lips or offer a small puréed dollop on their tray, so they can explore with their hands before smelling or tasting it. Never put anything directly in your baby's mouth without their approval.

FOLLOW YOUR BABY'S GUIDANCE. Some babies may want to eat a lot, some may choose a teaspoon, and others may not be interested at all. All are totally acceptable.

REINTRODUCE REJECTED FOODS SEVERAL TIMES. If you offer rejected foods in different forms (purée, chunky, or a whole slice), they'll have more exposure, which increases the likelihood they will try it again and possibly like it.

AVOID WIPING YOUR BABY DOWN WHILE FEEDING. It might be tempting, but the less you wipe them down during mealtime, the more you can help them be explorative and less picky.

STOP FEEDING AS SOON AS YOUR BABY LOSES INTEREST. It's usually made clear when they start to engage their environmental surroundings instead of the food. By encouraging "one more bite," you hinder their ability to be more self-intuitive and recognize when they've had enough.

The Food Adventure Begins

After bone broth, there are a few different ways you can go. You can introduce fruits and veggies, or meat. Avocado, banana, carrots, and sweet potatoes are great low-allergenic first fruits and vegetables to offer your little one. You can opt to offer savory over sweet produce first, just as long as you are offering a variety. Bananas and other tropical fruits are generally okay in the first month or two of having solids.

Be mindful that babies need an iron boost around 6 to 9 months, so I recommend introducing a red meat, which contains more iron than vegetables at this age. Red meat's iron levels (3.3mg iron per 100g) are significantly greater than vegetable offerings such as carrots (0.6mg iron per 100g). Simply incorporate the meat alongside the other foods on your baby's food journey. Ground beef or another iron-rich red meat purée is a good choice to start with.

Superfoods for Baby

If you're feeling adventurous and looking to take your nourishing food game to the next level, consider offering some of these superfoods to your baby. They can be offered in the first couple months of starting solids.

- Soft-boiled egg yolk (make sure to only offer the yolk since most inflammatory and allergic reactions come from the white)
- Liver pâté (this pairs well with a root vegetable like carrot or sweet potato)
- Bone marrow (try combining it with a mashed banana)
- Fish roe (try mixing with egg yolk or a puréed carrot)
- Sauerkraut brine (the juice in a quality sauerkraut can contain more probiotic organisms than a store-bought probiotic)

In recent years, liver has become a popular first food for babies for two reasons: It's rich in heme iron (8.8mg of iron per 100g compared to 3.3mg per 100g in red meat) and it's easily digestible, being an organ meat. In the 1950s, Gerber even offered liver because it had high nutritional offerings and a complex variety of B vitamins. Liver pâté was one of the first foods for both of my kids, and they loved it. I encourage parents not to be limited by their own food biases. You may be surprised by your little one's palate, if you give it a shot! See Resources (page 234) for more guidance.

Food Allergies and Intolerances

It's not uncommon for first-time parents to confuse food allergies with food intolerances or sensitivities. A food allergy occurs when the body initiates an immune response to a food and can be life-threatening. The nine most common allergens include:

- Cow's milk
- Wheat (gluten)
- Egg
- Soy
- Peanuts
- Tree nuts
- Shellfish
- Fish
- Sesame

A food intolerance or sensitivity occurs when the body has a difficult time digesting a particular food, often experiencing gas, belly pain, constipation, or diarrhea. Gassy foods that can be mistaken for an intolerance include beans, cruciferous vegetables (broccoli, cauliflower), and onions. These foods aren't bad and shouldn't be avoided. Just keep in mind if your baby seems uncomfortable after eating them, it's because they are gassy foods, not because your baby's intolerant.

Mild/Moderate Symptoms of an Allergic Reaction:

- A new rash
- Irritability
- Anxiousness
- Belly pain
- Itching
- Hives around the mouth or face
- Diaper rash around the anus

Severe Symptoms of an Allergic Reaction:

- Lip swelling
- Vomiting
- Hives or welts all over the body
- Face or tongue swelling
- Trouble breathing
- Wheezing
- Coughing
- Change in skin color to pale blue
- Dizziness
- Sudden tiredness or loss of consciousness

A baby's microbiome is always evolving and changing in the first three years of life. Therefore, a complete food allergen panel (test) under age 2 is not recommended. This can lead to over-diagnosis of a food allergy and unnecessary food restrictions. After year one, many babies seem to "outgrow" food sensitivities that present in the form of eczema or other mild reactions. You'll want to cut that food out for a couple months, focus on gut-healing foods, but then reintroduce it to see how they respond. Note that this reintroduction should not be done for foods that initiated a severe allergic reaction such as anaphylaxis. Babies that have a mild allergic response to foods in mom's breast milk may benefit from their breastfeeding mom taking a specific strain of a prebiotic called beta-glucan, which can help the immune reaction. Sometimes reactions like eczema resolve themselves over time. Oftentimes it can be more stubborn, in which case it can be helpful to work with your health care provider for guidance. There are even targeted probiotics you can give directly to babies to help with eczema or breaking down histamine (which causes eczema to show).

FOOD ALLERGY PREVENTION

In 2019, the American Academy of Pediatrics (AAP) released new guidelines for preventing food allergies and introducing the common allergens. They recommend:

1. An early, intentional introduction of allergens can help reduce your baby's food allergy risk.

2. Introduce the most common allergens like peanut, egg, and cow's milk when your baby is 6 to 11 months old, even if they are at a low or high risk for food allergies. (Peanuts can be offered ground or as nut butter. Egg yolk at 6 to 10 months; egg white at 9 to 12 months. Kefir or plain, full-fat organic yogurt can be given to a baby around 9 to 10 months, beginning with kefir preferably.)

3. Families with a peanut allergy history and/or severe eczema* should introduce peanuts to their baby by 6 months. (Don't stress if your baby hasn't started solids yet! This is just a recommendation.)

4. Breastfeeding alone is not guaranteed to prevent food allergies (though they get traces of the common allergens through mother's milk). Breastfeeding may help prevent eczema.

5. Feeding your baby hydrolyzed formula will not minimize your baby's risk for a food allergy.

Eczema is the greatest risk factor for developing a childhood food allergy. If your baby has eczema, I recommend working with a nurse coach to help reverse and reduce this likelihood.

If you have a family history of a food allergy, check with your pediatrician about your child's specific needs before making any food introductions.

FOODS TO AVOID
IN THE FIRST YEAR

There are plenty of foods baby can eat in the first year, but here are some they should avoid for a variety of reasons. If there is a family history of a food allergy, check with your pediatrician on introducing that food (see Food Allergy Prevention, page 52).

- Honey
- Raw carrots or vegetables (hard to digest in addition to choking hazard)
- Popcorn
- Whole seeds or nuts
- High-sodium foods (smoked or cured foods, certain cheese like feta)
- Hot dogs or sausages (the shape is a choking hazard)
- High-mercury fish (swordfish, tuna, shark)
- Corn
- Water, juice, or soda (water should only be given in small amounts; see page 63)
- Processed/refined sugar
- Pre-packaged foods or snacks from a box
- Teething biscuits (for healthier options, see Teething Foods, page 56)
- Grains, beans, or legumes that have not been soaked/sprouted
- Pasteurized cow's milk (see Introducing Milk at 12 Months, page 163)

Dairy in other forms, such as full-fat yogurt and cheese may be introduced before age 1. Whole nuts, seeds, carrots, popcorn, and grapes are a choking hazard and should be avoided until age 4, according to the American Association of Pediatrics. These foods can be offered in different forms such as quartering grapes, grating carrots, and offering nuts in the form of nut butters mixed into foods.

Introducing New Food

When introducing new foods, including common allergens, it's important to consider both the wellness of your child and the amount of time you need to watch your child after introducing the allergen. Here are some guidelines to follow when introducing new foods, including common allergens:

- Introduce new foods only when your baby is feeling well. Avoid the introduction of an allergen if your baby is showing signs of belly stress.
- Make sure you're at home and present for the introduction, not elsewhere eating out or leaving the baby in the care of another person.
- Offer your baby a new food in the morning. Avoid feeding within 4 hours of naptime or bedtime, since it can take a few hours to show a reaction and you want to be alert to any changes.
- Offer a small taste, about ¼ teaspoon, of the new food or common allergen. Wait for 15 to 30 minutes and monitor for a response. If baby has no reaction, offer another ¼ to 2 teaspoons.
- Give your baby your undivided attention for a few hours after the introduction, keeping an eye on baby's stool and mood.
- Wait 3 days after introducing a new food before continuing to offer the food. Monitor your baby for any reactions for 3 days after the introduction.

Gagging and Choking

Choking or gagging are quite different, though both can feel like a scary experience for you and your baby. Understanding their causes and differences can help you react appropriately to assist your baby. It can be lifesaving (and give you peace of mind) to take a first-aid and CPR course to learn how to respond to an obstructed airway and other emergencies that can occur.

GAGGING

Gagging is a safety reflex that babies have, and it does not require intervention. Gagging is usually accompanied by a red face, frustration, coughing, and an effort to spit out a food. It is normal for your baby to gag or make funny faces when experiencing the texture and tastes of new foods for the first time. If the texture makes them gag, you can make the purée smoother by adding a little bit of breast milk, water, bone broth, or formula.

If your baby starts to gag or has too much food in their mouth, they may need your help. Show them what to do by sticking your own tongue out several times, repeating this gesture while saying "ah."

CHOKING

Choking occurs when the airway is blocked, and this requires immediate intervention. Choking presents with silence (so no coughing or crying), blueness around the lips or the face, and possible loss of consciousness. You can help prevent choking by supervising eating, so that you're available for early intervention if needed, and by cutting round foods (grapes, tomatoes, etc.) into quarters rather than in half. Never place your hands into the mouth of a choking child, as it may further lodge the object and cause more distress.

What to do if your baby is choking:

1. Lay your baby face-down along your forearm (you can also use your lap or thigh).
2. In the same arm that is holding baby, support their jaw while holding their chest in your hand.
3. Place their head lower than their body, allowing gravity to help.
4. Give up to 5 short and forceful blows between their shoulder blades using the palm of your free hand.
5. If you see the foreign object in their mouth, gently use one finger to sweep it out.

Good Eating Can Be Fun!

Although we focus on all the guidelines and "right things" to do when it comes to feeding your baby, let's not lose sight of how much fun feeding your little one can be. Playing, exploring, squishing, smashing, licking, making a mess—it's all part of the adventure! Of course, with this part, get ready for a few extra baths, too.

As messy as mealtime may be, you can also encourage self-feeding to help develop independence, self-confidence, and a broader sense of food texture and taste experiences. Self-feeding also prevents picky eaters. If you want to offer a spoon, you can easily pre-load it for them to practice. If you want to forgo, it's totally fine to just let them use their hands.

When families interact with food in a positive manner, this can help your baby develop a positive relationship with food. Even if your baby has a "picky phase," it's usually short-lived, so don't sweat it, and don't be afraid to re-introduce those rejected foods another time.

TEETHING FOODS

The discomfort of teething can turn your little one off of food, or trigger a strong urge to chew on more textures. Counterpressure on the gums feels good to a baby with incoming teeth, so try offering some of these easy go-to teething foods—always with supervision:

- Single foods that have been chilled in the refrigerator (such as carrot, cucumber, celery) or frozen (such as a green bean).
- Frozen breast milk or coconut milk ice cube in a silicone teething pouch.
- Frozen fruit chunks like mango or pineapple in a silicone teething pouch.
- Baby ice pop—just blend their favorite fruits or veggies and freeze in ice pop molds.

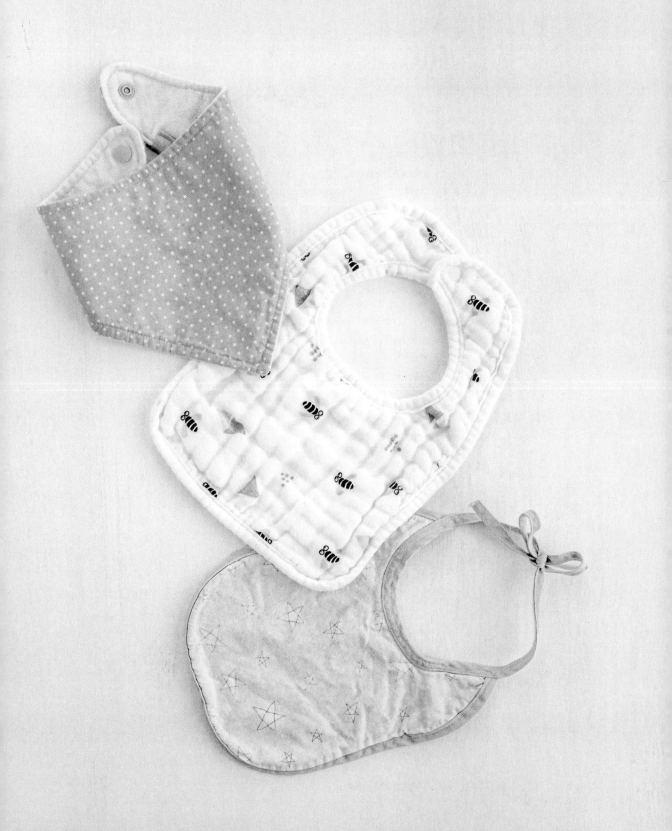

POSITIVE FOOD LANGUAGE

Many parents often say common well-intended phrases about food such as "Broccoli is good for you" or "Sugar is bad." They may even begin to stereotype their kid's relationship to food, like, "They're so picky; don't bother giving them that." By enhancing your language around food, you can create an environment of positive food talk and energy.

Restricting foods (all forms of sugar, for example) can lead to overconsumption in the future, so just be mindful with the language you use around it. Talking about how "bad" a food is can make it more tempting! Of course, kids are impulsive and we have to be the voice of reason when it comes to offering foods. Our job is simply to offer healthy options and portions, while allowing them to choose what and how much they want to eat. Instead of demonizing certain things like sugar, we can teach them the facts. A good fact to share might be: *Sugar offers quick energy, but then wears off quickly. Or, Sugar does not feed our "good bugs" in our bellies (aka good bacteria).*

Here are some other phrases to consider:

Common Food Phrase	What Children Think	Positive Talk/Action to Help Them Understand
"It's dinner time and you have to eat."	Even though my body is saying it's not hungry, I should still eat because my parent said I have to.	"It's a long time from now until morning, so now is the time to eat if you are hungry."
"You didn't eat enough. Take a few more bites."	Parents are better judges at knowing when I am full.	"Listen to your body and eat if you are hungry. It's a while before snack time/next meal."
"Good job!" after eating all their food/vegetables	How much I eat is more important than listening to my body.	"You always do a good job eating when you listen to your body."
"She's so picky; she only eats a couple foods."	Something must be wrong with me.	"We are trying new foods together!"

Common Food Phrase	What Children Think	Positive Talk/Action to Help Them Understand
"Your sister ate all her food; don't you want to?"	My sister must be a better eater than me.	"My kids like different types of food."
"Don't waste your time giving him any of that salad; he won't eat it."	If I don't like something the first time I try it, they won't try to make me eat it again.	"I will put a little of the salad on the side of your plate, and if you want to try it, you can."
"If you finish your fish, I will give you a cookie."	Cookies are better than fish.	Rather than bribes, try surprising your child with a dessert (like a few dark chocolate chips) and serve it alongside a meal.
"Sugar is bad for you; it makes your teeth rot."	I must be bad if I eat sugar.	"We always brush our teeth after eating sugar."
"Chocolate chips aren't a healthy breakfast."	Sometimes chocolate chips are in the special waffles we make together on Saturdays, so are those not healthy?	"I love chocolate chips, too. Maybe we can have some later today."

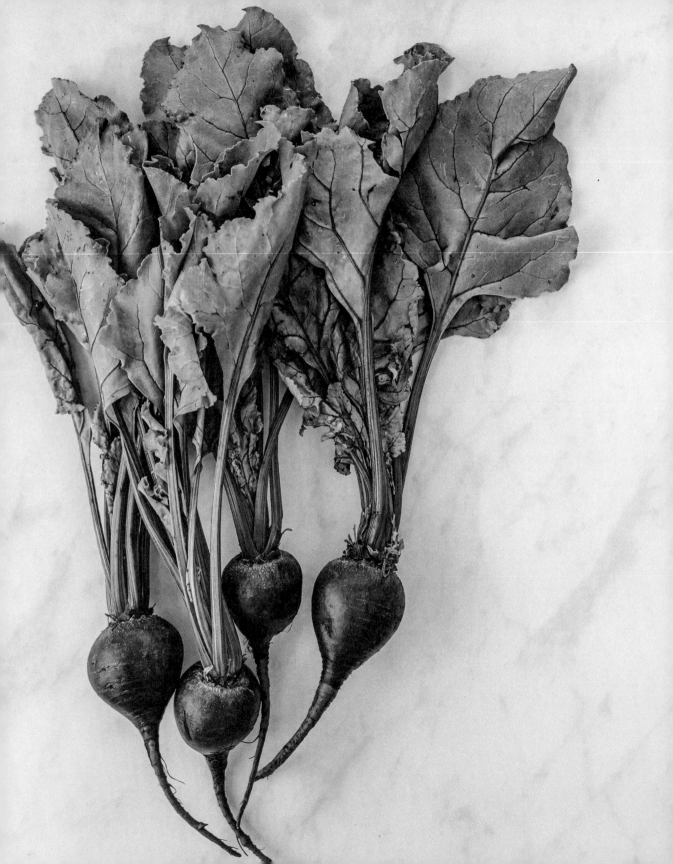

Five

Single-Ingredient Foods

6 TO 8 MONTHS

The recipes in this chapter are single-ingredient, to introduce one food at a time. Feed your baby just one new food and wait 3 days before feeding again to monitor for an allergic reaction (see page 54). Once the foods are tolerated without any reaction, feel free to move on to another food. Babies may not eat too much of a solid food when introduced, but don't let this discourage you. If they reject a food, be sure to re-introduce it in a different way (puréed versus soft-cooked). It's all new to them, so don't give up on a food if it's not "love at first bite." Also, a few of the recipes call for coconut oil and/or spices. You can always choose to introduce the food by itself before adding the oil or spice called for in the recipe if you wish to be extra-careful about identifying the source of any possible reaction.

In this chapter, many of the fruits are offered around 7 to 8 months. That is intentional, as the first 2 to 3 weeks of feeding should be bone broth, followed by avocado, vegetables, and iron-rich meats. Avocado, banana, carrots, and sweet potatoes are great low-allergenic first fruits and vegetables to offer your little one after the bone broth. You can opt to offer savory over sweet produce first, but remember to offer a variety. Bananas and other tropical fruits are generally okay in the first month or two of having solids.

WHAT TO EXPECT

Even as your baby starts solids, their main source of nutrition will still be breast milk or formula. After offering a starter food like bone broth to prepare baby's gut, you can offer puréed, soft-cooked, mashed, or specifically sliced soft foods. The consistency of the purées should be thin and watery at first. You can add a splash of breast milk, formula, bone broth, or filtered water to any of the recipes to thin them out. Over time, you can increase the texture to make it a little lumpier.

How Much to Feed
1 to 2 tablespoons. As the weeks go by, follow baby's lead and increase their serving size to about ¼ cup.

When to Feed
Once per day, about mid-morning, after feeding breast milk or formula earlier in the morning

What to Drink
For ages 6 to 12 months, it's okay to offer daily 2 to 3 ounces of water **max** in a cup. This will allow them to practice and play while they are eating solids. Never offer water as a fluid replacement for breast milk or formula, which should still be the primary source of nutrition and fluid in the first 12 months.

First-Time Parent Tip

Before puréeing any of the fruit in the following recipes, reserve some of the fruit, chop into smaller pieces, and freeze individually. Add the frozen fruit to a mesh or silicone feeder as a teething treat.

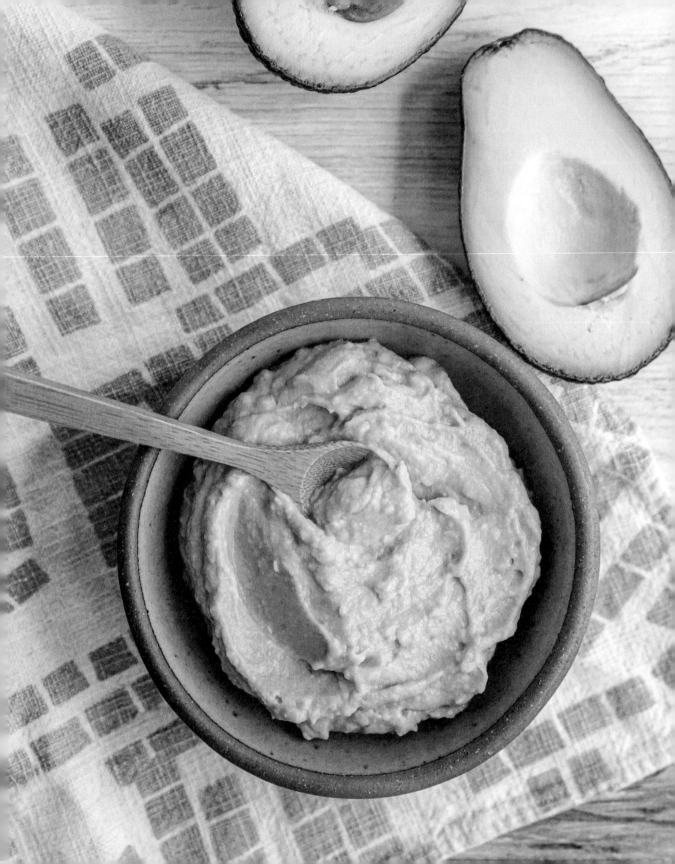

FRUIT RECIPES

Avocado Mash

PREP TIME: 5 minutes
DAIRY-FREE • **GLUTEN-FREE** • **NUT-FREE** • **VEGAN** • **VEGETARIAN**

Avocado was the first thing I served my babies after giving them bone broth. High in monounsaturated fats, avocados are a mild, creamy, brain-boosting first food. To choose a good avocado, look for one that is soft on the outside. Then gently remove the brown stem (if there is one) to make sure it's green underneath. If it's brown, it may be overripe. **MAKES ½ CUP**

½ ripe avocado, pitted and peeled

1 tablespoon filtered water

In a small bowl, combine the avocado and water. Using a fork, mash and mix. For first bites, the consistency should be thin and easy to slide off a spoon.

Storage: Keep the mashed avocado in a glass jar in the refrigerator up to 3 days. Not suitable for freezing.

Tip: Instead of water, you can also try using breast milk, formula, or, for a non-vegetarian version, bone broth.

Mashed Banana

PREP TIME: 5 minutes
DAIRY-FREE • **GLUTEN-FREE** • **NUT-FREE** • **VEGAN** • **VEGETARIAN**

Perfect for babies around 6 ½ months old, bananas are high in amylase, which aids digestion. Its creamy, mild texture and slightly sweet flavor make this food a home run with most babies and toddlers. As a bonus, it's one of the least expensive whole foods money can buy. **MAKES ½ CUP**

½ ripe banana, peeled

1 tablespoon filtered water

In a small bowl, combine the banana and water. Using a fork, mash and mix. For first bites, the consistency should be thin and easy to slide off a spoon.

Storage: Keep the mashed banana in a glass jar in the refrigerator for 1 to 2 days. Not suitable for freezing.

Tip: Instead of water, you can also try using breast milk, formula, or, for a non-vegetarian version, bone broth.

Soft-Cooked Apple

PREP TIME: 10 to 15 minutes **COOK TIME:** 10 to 15 minutes

FREEZER-FRIENDLY • BLW • DAIRY-FREE • GLUTEN-FREE • NUT-FREE • VEGAN • VEGETARIAN

You can introduce cooked apples when baby is 6 ½ to 7 months old. At this age, cooking fruits and veggies is the best way to maximize their nutrient absorption and digestion. You can make this recipe as a purée or serve it in very soft cooked pieces that are easily picked up and "mashable" between the gums (typically after 8 to 10 months, when they've developed the pincer grasp). Consider mixing tart apples like Granny Smith with sweeter ones like Gala or Honeycrisp. **MAKES ABOUT SIXTEEN 1-OUNCE FREEZER CUBES**

3 tablespoons coconut oil (optional)

1 ¼ pounds apples (4 apples), peeled, cored, and cut into ¼-inch dice

Filtered water

1 In a medium saucepan, heat the coconut oil over low heat (if using). (Before making this recipe, you can introduce coconut oil by itself to test for any possible reaction.)

2 Add the apples and cover with about ½ inch filtered water. Cover with a lid, bring to a simmer, and cook for 5 to 10 minutes, or until very soft. Remove from the heat. Let cool for a few minutes with the lid off. Serve as is, or transfer to a blender and purée to your desired consistency.

Storage: Divide into ice cube trays, freeze overnight, then transfer to an airtight zip-top bag or glass container. Freeze for up to 6 months.

Pairings: Apples pair well with sage, cinnamon, nutmeg, fennel, or ginger. Add just a small pinch before serving or purée-ing. They also pair really well with coconut cream; serve alongside whole pieces or mixed into a purée.

Soft-Cooked Pear

PREP TIME: 10 to 15 minutes   **COOK TIME:** 10 to 15 minutes

FREEZER-FRIENDLY · BLW · **DAIRY-FREE** · **GLUTEN-FREE** · **NUT-FREE** · **VEGAN** · **VEGETARIAN**

Another great first food to introduce at 6 ½ to 7 months of age, pear delights with its mild, sweet flavor. Pears soften and sweeten up as they ripen, and you may want to hold on to your pears until they're ripe before cooking. This recipe is prepared similarly to the Soft-Cooked Apple (page 66). You can make pears as a purée or cooked in very soft pieces that baby can pick up and mash between the gums (typically after 8 to 10 months, when they've developed the pincer grasp). Consider combining a sweet pear like Anjou or Bartlett with a crispier Asian pear. In addition to their nutritional value, pears are also great for relieving constipation in your little one. MAKES ABOUT SIXTEEN 1-OUNCE FREEZER CUBES

3 tablespoons coconut oil (optional)

1 ½ pounds ripe pears (3 to 4 medium pears), peeled, cored, and cut into ¼-inch dice

Filtered water

1   In a medium saucepan, heat the coconut oil over low heat (if using). (Before making this recipe, you can introduce coconut oil by itself to test for any possible reaction.)

2   Add the pears and cover with about ½ inch filtered water. Cover with a lid, bring to a simmer, and cook for 5 to 10 minutes, or until very soft. Remove from the heat. Let cool for a few minutes with the lid off. Serve as is, or transfer to a blender, and purée to your desired consistency.

Storage: Divide into ice cube trays, freeze overnight, and transfer to an airtight zip-top bag or glass container. Freeze for up to 6 months.

Pairings: Pears go well with cinnamon, anise, fennel, or ginger. Add just a small pinch before serving or puréeing. They also pair really well with coconut cream; serve alongside whole pieces or mixed into a purée.

Soft-Cooked Cherries

PREP TIME: 15 to 25 minutes **COOK TIME:** 5 to 10 minutes

FREEZER-FRIENDLY · **DAIRY-FREE** · **GLUTEN-FREE** · **NUT-FREE** · **VEGAN** · **VEGETARIAN**

Sweet little cherries are a food powerhouse! They carry loads of antioxidants and anti-inflammatory and vitamin-rich nutrients, making them protective for your little one's immune system. They even help regulate melatonin, making sleep cycles more regular. Full of vitamins C and K, fiber, and potassium, cherries are also delicious. A win-win! They are best served pitted, cooked, and either puréed or smashed (around 6 to 7 months of age), or raw, pitted, sliced, and quartered (around 9 months of age). **MAKES ABOUT SIXTEEN 1-OUNCE FREEZER CUBES**

3 tablespoons coconut oil (optional)

1 ½ pounds cherries (about 3 cups), stemmed and pitted

Filtered water

1   In a medium saucepan, heat the coconut oil over low heat (if using). (Before making this recipe, you can introduce coconut oil by itself to test for any possible reaction.)

2   Add the cherries and cover with about ½ inch filtered water. Cover with a lid, bring to a simmer, and cook for about 5 minutes, or until very soft. Remove from the heat. Let cool for a few minutes with the lid off.

3   Smash each cherry between two fingers before serving, or transfer to a blender, and purée to your desired consistency.

Storage: Divide into ice cube trays, freeze overnight, and transfer to an airtight zip-top bag or glass container. Freeze for up to 6 months.

Pairings: Cherries taste good with almonds, bananas, walnuts, cinnamon, and even thyme. Try grinding one of those nuts and sprinkling it on top of the cherries, after cherries have been introduced and pending no allergic reaction.

Peach Purée

PREP TIME: 10 to 15 minutes **COOK TIME:** 10 to 15 minutes

FREEZER-FRIENDLY · **DAIRY-FREE** · **GLUTEN-FREE** · **NUT-FREE** · **VEGAN** · **VEGETARIAN**

Is it possible to not love a juicy, sweet, in-season peach? Peaches are the perfect seasonal fruit, bright and tasty, and loaded with beta-carotene, vitamins C and A, fiber, and potassium. Peaches can typically be introduced to your baby at 7 to 8 months of age. Peaches are on the Dirty Dozen list (page 12), making them a good choice for your organic dollar. **MAKES ABOUT SIXTEEN 1-OUNCE FREEZER CUBES**

3 tablespoons coconut oil (optional)

1 ½ pounds ripe peaches (3 to 4 peaches), pitted, peeled, and cut into ¼-inch dice

1   In a medium saucepan, heat the coconut oil over low heat (if using). (Before making this recipe, you can introduce coconut oil by itself to test for any possible reaction.)

2   Add the peaches and cover with about ½ inch filtered water. Cover with a lid, bring to a simmer, and cook for 5 to 10 minutes, or until very soft. Remove from the heat. Let cool for a few minutes with the lid off. Transfer to a blender, and purée to your desired consistency.

Storage: Divide into ice cube trays, freeze overnight, and transfer to an airtight zip-top bag or glass container. Freeze for up to 6 months.

Pairings: Peaches taste good with almonds, hazelnuts, ginger, clove, cinnamon, or even basil. Try grinding one of those nuts and sprinkling it on top of the peaches, after peaches have been introduced and pending no allergic reaction.

FRUIT RECIPES

Papaya Purée

PREP TIME: 5 minutes
FREEZER-FRIENDLY · DAIRY-FREE · GLUTEN-FREE · NUT-FREE · VEGAN · VEGETARIAN

I love papaya for babies because of its smooth texture and mild taste. Papaya is one of the easiest fruits to prepare and serve as a smooth purée or mash. They are rich in special enzymes, essentially pre-digested for your baby. They also contain vitamins A and C along with magnesium, making them another good food for easing constipation. Expand your fruit horizons and offer papaya to baby at 7 to 8 months of age. **MAKES ABOUT SIXTEEN 1-OUNCE FREEZER CUBES**

1 ½ cups diced fresh papaya (about 1 ½ papayas)

Put the papaya in a blender or food processor, and purée.

Storage: Divide into ice cube trays, freeze overnight, and transfer to an airtight zip-top bag or glass container. Freeze for up to 6 months.

Tip: Purée with other fruits like mango (once all have been introduced and pending no reaction), freeze into cubes, and serve thawed like little fruit sorbets.

Pineapple Purée

PREP TIME: 5 minutes
FREEZER-FRIENDLY · DAIRY-FREE · GLUTEN-FREE · NUT-FREE · VEGAN · VEGETARIAN

Besides its bright color and flavor, pineapple contains a natural anti-inflammatory compound called bromelain. Bromelain also aids in digestion, making it a perfect food for babies starting solids. Since pineapple can be a little stringy and firm in some places, chop and purée it with a small amount of liquid before puréeing the rest. Serve it around 8 months of age. Note: Pineapple is a higher-acidity food, and can cause a rash around the mouth or diaper area. If your baby is sensitive or already experiencing a rash, wait until they are closer to 9 to 10 months of age. **MAKES ABOUT SIXTEEN 1-OUNCE FREEZER CUBES**

1 ½ cups fresh pineapple chunks (about ½ small pineapple)

Put the pineapple in a blender or food processor, and purée.

Storage: Divide into ice cube trays, freeze overnight, and transfer to an airtight zip-top bag or glass container. Freeze for up to 6 months.

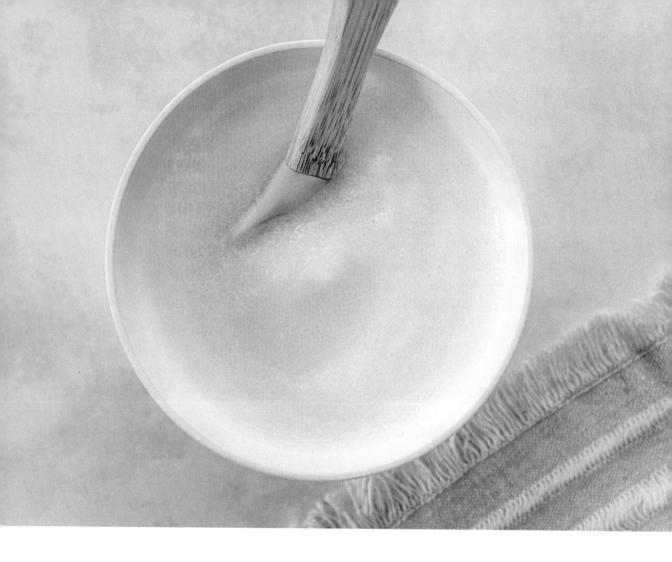

Tip: If the pineapple is too stringy, consider cooking it for a few minutes and then puréeing.

Pairings: Purée with other fruits like mango or papaya (once all have been introduced and pending no reaction), freeze into cubes, and serve thawed like little fruit sorbets.

Kiwi Mash or Purée

PREP TIME: 5 minutes
FREEZER-FRIENDLY · DAIRY-FREE · GLUTEN-FREE · NUT-FREE · VEGAN · VEGETARIAN

Kiwis are good for babies because even though they have tiny seeds, the seeds are soft and edible. Kiwi is rich in vitamins A and C and high in potassium, fiber, and folate. Kiwi is not a common allergen, but it is acidic and can prompt redness around the mouth, or on the bottom after a bowel movement. Offer to your baby around 8 months of age, unless they are already battling a diaper rash, in which case you may want to wait until they are closer to 10 months of age. MAKES ABOUT ⅓ CUP

1 kiwi, peeled and quartered

Put the kiwi in a small bowl, and using a fork, mash. Or, transfer to a blender, and purée.

Storage: Keep leftover kiwi in a glass container in the refrigerator for up to 3 days.

Cantaloupe Mash

PREP TIME: 5 minutes
FREEZER-FRIENDLY · DAIRY-FREE · GLUTEN-FREE · NUT-FREE · VEGAN · VEGETARIAN

Rich in beta-carotene, cantaloupe is great for your little one's eyes, skin, and hair. It's also a juicy and tasty treat, so roll up your sleeves and enjoy this smooth melon with your babe! The rind can hold bacteria, so be sure to wash and scrub the cantaloupe with clean water before cutting into it, as the knife can transfer the bacteria from the rind onto the fruit. MAKES ¼ CUP

¼ cup chopped cantaloupe

Put the cantaloupe in a small bowl, and using a fork, mash.

Storage: Keep leftover melon in a glass container in the refrigerator for up to 3 days.

Tip: Choose a cantaloupe that smells sweet at the stem. Always wash melons before cutting them, since they grow on the ground and can contain bacteria. You can also offer this as a slice rather than a mash. At 7 to 8 months of age, offer it cut into slices about the thickness of a ruler.

Watermelon Mash

PREP TIME: 5 minutes

FREEZER-FRIENDLY · DAIRY-FREE · GLUTEN-FREE · NUT-FREE · VEGAN · VEGETARIAN

That pinky-red flesh of watermelon is rich in a powerful antioxidant called lycopene. In addition to watermelon's health benefits, it's just plain fun! Watermelon is at its ripest in late summer when it is high in water content, making it a refreshing treat for a hot day. It's easy to prepare, and it's almost always a hit! MAKES ¼ CUP

¼ cup chopped watermelon

Put the watermelon in a small bowl, and using a fork, mash.

Storage: Keep leftover melon in a glass container in the refrigerator for up to 3 days.

Tip: Look for a seedless watermelon, which contains soft beige seeds rather than the hard black ones. A ripe watermelon usually has a big yellow spot on it. You can also offer this as a slice rather than a mash. At 7 to 8 months of age, offer it cut into slices about the thickness of a ruler.

Mango Purée

PREP TIME: 5 minutes

FREEZER-FRIENDLY · DAIRY-FREE · GLUTEN-FREE · NUT-FREE · VEGAN · VEGETARIAN

There's nothing more delicious than a ripe mango! Mangos are high in vitamins E and C, making them protective for your baby's immune system. They also are packed with vitamin A, important for baby's eye development. How to tell if a mango is ripe? It'll be reddish, yellow, or orange; give a little when you squeeze it; and smell fruity at the stem. There's an easy 45-second tutorial for how to cut a mango at mango.org. Serve this fruit at around 7 to 8 months of age. MAKES ABOUT SIXTEEN 1-OUNCE FREEZER CUBES

1 pound mangos, peeled, pitted, and cut into ½-inch dice or 1 (16-ounce) package of frozen mangos

Put the mango in a blender, and purée until smooth.

Storage: Divide into ice cube trays, freeze overnight, and transfer to an airtight zip-top bag or glass container. Freeze for up to 6 months. You can alternatively keep some of the purée in a glass jar in the refrigerator for up to 3 days.

Strawberry Purée

PREP TIME: 10 minutes **COOK TIME:** 10 minutes

FREEZER-FRIENDLY · **DAIRY-FREE** · **GLUTEN-FREE** · **NUT-FREE** · **VEGAN** · **VEGETARIAN**

Like many berries, strawberries are loaded with antioxidants and anti-inflammatory properties. Raw berries can be hard to digest for some babies, so at this age, cooking them is best until a couple months from now. You can certainly try offering raw berries (safely, of course), but this favorite breakfast treat is more easily digestible when cooked. It also provides optimal nutrient absorption this way. Strawberries are a good place to spend your organic dollar, as conventionally grown strawberries are among the produce most contaminated by pesticides. **MAKES ABOUT SIXTEEN 1-OUNCE FREEZER CUBES**

2 cups fresh or frozen strawberries

2 tablespoons coconut oil (optional)

Filtered water

1. Hull the strawberries if using fresh: Using a paring knife, cut in a circle around the green, leafy stem to remove.

2. In a small saucepan, heat the coconut oil over medium heat (if using). (Before making this recipe, you can introduce coconut oil by itself to test for any possible reaction.)

3. Add the berries and cover with about ½ inch filtered water. Cover with a lid, and cook for about 5 minutes, or until soft and warm. Remove from the heat. Let cool for a few minutes with the lid off. Transfer to a blender, and purée to your desired consistency.

Storage: Divide into ice cube trays, freeze overnight, and transfer to an airtight zip-top bag or glass container. Freeze for up to 6 months. You can alternatively save some in a glass jar in the refrigerator for up to 3 days and divide the rest to freeze.

Tip: You could alternatively serve this as a mash rather than a purée. If it is too thin, you can mix this into another food your baby has already been introduced to. And if you're comfortable with dairy, you can use ghee or grass-fed butter instead of coconut oil.

Pairings: You can serve strawberries alongside coconut cream for a tasty treat once it has been introduced, pending no reaction.

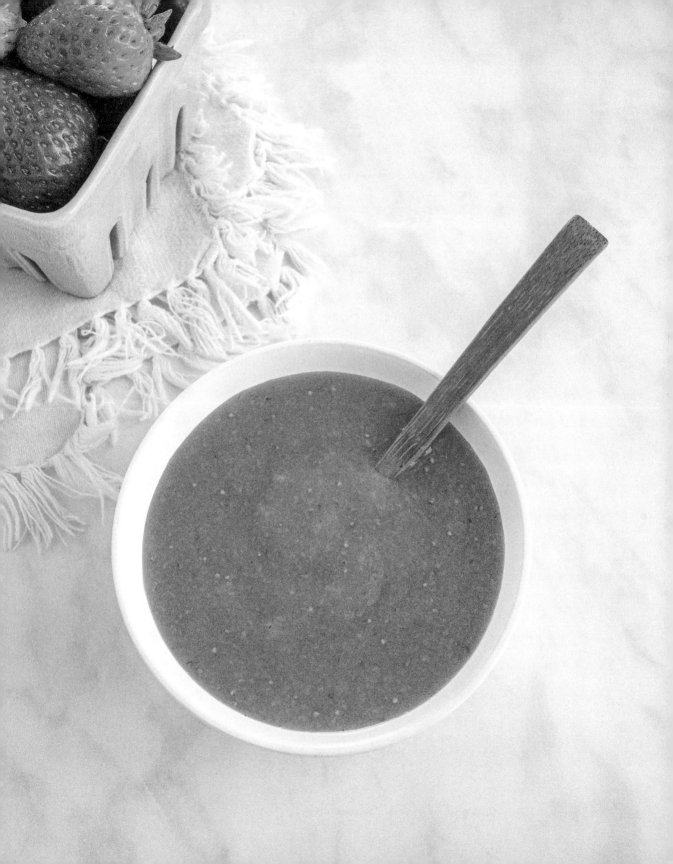

Mashed Sweet Potato

PREP TIME: 10 minutes **COOK TIME:** 15 to 20 minutes
FREEZER-FRIENDLY · **DAIRY-FREE** · **GLUTEN-FREE** · **NUT-FREE** · **VEGAN** · **VEGETARIAN**

Root vegetables like sweet potatoes provide complex carbs for growing littles. These macronutrients give their body the energy they need for the day's adventures! Complex carbs are preferred over simple carbs because they help maintain level blood sugars. Sweet potatoes, in particular, are rich in beta-carotene and fiber and have a smooth texture when mashed.

MAKES ABOUT SIXTEEN 1-OUNCE FREEZER CUBES

2 large sweet potatoes, peeled and cut into 1-inch dice

¼ to ½ cup filtered water, plus more as needed

1 to 2 tablespoons coconut oil (optional)

1   In a medium pot, combine the sweet potatoes and water. Cover with a lid, bring to a simmer over medium-low heat, and cook for 10 to 15 minutes, or until very soft. Add a splash of water if it starts to look dry. Remove from the heat. Using a slotted spoon, transfer to a bowl.

2   Add the coconut oil (if using) and mash. (Before making this recipe, you can introduce coconut oil by itself to test for any possible reaction.)

3   Add the cooking liquid from the pot until you reach your desired consistency. You can also purée the sweet potatoes with the cooking liquid in a blender.

Storage: Divide into ice cube trays, freeze overnight, and transfer to an airtight zip-top bag or glass container. Freeze for up to 6 months. You can alternatively save some a glass jar in the refrigerator for up to 3 days and divide the rest to freeze.

Tip: If you're comfortable with dairy, you can use ghee or grass-fed butter instead of coconut oil. For a non-vegetarian version, try using bone broth instead of water.

Pumpkin Purée

PREP TIME: 10 minutes **COOK TIME:** 20 minutes

FREEZER-FRIENDLY · **DAIRY-FREE** · **GLUTEN-FREE** · **NUT-FREE** · **VEGAN** · **VEGETARIAN**

Pumpkins are most available in fall through early winter. Stock up on them because they last quite a while if stored in a cool, dark, dry place. If you don't have a pumpkin or are making this recipe out of season, you can grab a bag of frozen pumpkin already seeded and chopped. Packed with vitamins A and C, pumpkins are pretty to look at and good for your little one's eyes and immune system. **MAKES ABOUT SIXTEEN 1-OUNCE FREEZER CUBES**

1 pound pumpkin, peeled, seeded, and cut into ½-inch dice (about 1 ½ cups)

¼ to ½ cup filtered water, plus more to thin to desired consistency

1 to 2 tablespoons coconut oil (optional)

1   In a medium pot, combine the pumpkin and water. Cover with a lid, bring to a simmer over medium-low heat, and cook for about 15 minutes, or until very soft. Remove from the heat. Transfer to a blender.

2   Add the coconut oil (if using) and purée, adding more water to thin to your desired consistency. (Before making this recipe, you can introduce coconut oil by itself to test for any possible reaction.)

Storage: Divide into ice cube trays, freeze overnight, and transfer to an airtight zip-top bag or glass container. Freeze for up to 6 months. You can alternatively save some in a glass jar in the refrigerator for up to 3 days and divide the rest to freeze.

Tip: Always wash pumpkins before cutting them, since they grow on the ground and can contain bacteria. If you're comfortable with dairy, you can use ghee or grass-fed butter instead of coconut oil. And for a non-vegetarian version, try using bone broth instead of water.

VEGGIE RECIPES

Butternut Squash Purée

PREP TIME: 10 minutes **COOK TIME:** 20 minutes
FREEZER-FRIENDLY · **DAIRY-FREE** · **GLUTEN-FREE** · **NUT-FREE** · **VEGAN** · **VEGETARIAN**

Butternut squash (and other winter squash) are most available late summer through winter. They can last up to a few months if stored in a cool, dark, dry place. If you don't have a butternut squash or are making this recipe out of season, you can grab a bag of frozen butternut squash, which is already nicely seeded and chopped. Packed with vitamins A and C, butternut squash is good for your little one's eyes and immune system. As baby grows, they can enjoy butternut squash prepared in other delicious ways that the whole family will enjoy, such as roasted and in soups. **MAKES ABOUT SIXTEEN 1-OUNCE FREEZER CUBES**

1 ½ pounds butternut squash, peeled, seeded, and cut into ½-inch dice

¼ to ½ cup filtered water, plus more to thin to desired consistency

1 to 2 tablespoons coconut oil (optional)

1   In a medium pot, combine the squash and water. Cover with a lid, bring to a simmer over medium-low heat, and cook for about 15 minutes, or until very soft. Remove from the heat. Transfer to a blender.

2   Add the coconut oil (if using) and purée, adding more water to thin to your desired consistency. (Before making this recipe, you can introduce coconut oil by itself to test for any possible reaction.)

Storage: Divide into ice cube trays, freeze overnight, and transfer to an airtight zip-top bag or glass container. Freeze for up to 6 months. You can alternatively save some in a glass jar in the refrigerator for up to 3 days and divide the rest to freeze.

Tip: Always wash squash before cutting them, since they grow on the ground and can contain bacteria. You could also use another variety of winter squash: acorn, kabocha, buttercup, or delicata, to name a few. If you're comfortable with dairy, you can use ghee or grass-fed butter instead of coconut oil. And for a non-vegetarian version, try using bone broth instead of water.

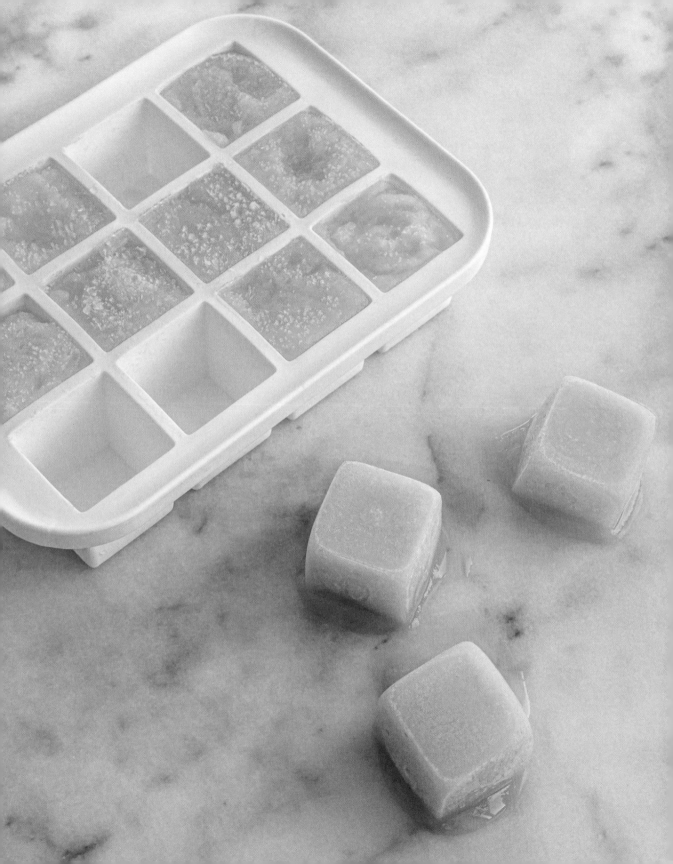

Soft-Cooked Zucchini

PREP TIME: 10 minutes **COOK TIME:** 10 minutes

FREEZER-FRIENDLY · BLW · DAIRY-FREE · GLUTEN-FREE · NUT-FREE · VEGAN · VEGETARIAN

Greens and raw salad are still too rough for baby's digestive system, so offering a little zucchini gives them a "green" boost while still maintaining that soft-cooked texture perfect for digestion. This recipe is super-easy and handy to offer as a soft-cooked finger food. **MAKES ABOUT SIXTEEN 1-OUNCE FREEZER CUBES**

3 small zucchini, peeled and cut into ¼-inch dice

¼ cup filtered water

1 to 2 tablespoons coconut oil (optional)

1   In a medium saucepan, combine the zucchini, water, and coconut oil (if using). (Before making this recipe, you can introduce coconut oil to test for any possible reaction.)

2   Cover with a lid, bring to a simmer over medium-low heat, and cook for 5 to 7 minutes, or until very soft. Remove from the heat.

Storage: Divide into ice cube trays, freeze overnight, and transfer to an airtight zip-top bag or glass container. Freeze for up to 6 months. You can alternatively save some in a glass jar in the refrigerator for up to 3 days and divide the rest to freeze.

Tip: You can also transfer the cooked zucchini to a blender, and purée, adding more water to reach your desired consistency. If you're comfortable with dairy, you can use ghee or grass-fed butter instead of coconut oil. And for a non-vegetarian version, try using bone broth instead of water.

Pairings: This recipe works with a dash of ground cumin or garlic powder.

Celery Purée

PREP TIME: 10 minutes COOK TIME: 10 minutes
FREEZER-FRIENDLY · DAIRY-FREE · GLUTEN-FREE · NUT-FREE · VEGAN · VEGETARIAN

Who would guess that celery could make a good first food? That's the beauty of purées! Since greens and raw salad are still too rough for your baby's digestive system, offering a little puréed celery gives them a "green" boost while still maintaining that soft-cooked texture perfect for digestion. Celery also delivers nerve protection, antioxidants, and immunity-boosting properties and is rich in vitamins and minerals. This is a good veggie to purchase organic, since it appears on the Dirty Dozen list (page 12). MAKES ABOUT 1 CUP

1 to 2 tablespoons coconut oil (optional)

4 celery stalks, cut into ½-inch pieces

¼ cup filtered water, plus more to thin to desired consistency

1 In a medium saucepan, heat the coconut oil over medium-low heat (if using). (Before making this recipe, you can introduce coconut oil by itself to test for any possible reaction.)

2 Add the celery and water. Cover with a lid, bring to a simmer, and cook for 5 to 7 minutes, or until very soft. Remove from the heat.

3 Transfer to a blender and purée, adding more water to thin to your desired consistency. Strain through a fine-mesh strainer to remove the stringy parts.

Storage: Divide into ice cube trays, freeze overnight, and transfer to an airtight zip-top bag or glass container. Freeze for up to 6 months. You can alternatively save some in a glass jar in the refrigerator for up to 3 days and divide the rest to freeze.

Tip: If you're comfortable with dairy, you can use ghee or grass-fed butter instead of coconut oil. And for a non-vegetarian version, try using bone broth instead of water.

Pairings: This recipe works with a dash of ground cumin or garlic powder.

Parsnip Purée

PREP TIME: 10 minutes **COOK TIME:** 10 minutes

FREEZER-FRIENDLY · **DAIRY-FREE** · **GLUTEN-FREE** · NUT-FREE · VEGAN · VEGETARIAN

Parsnips are an underutilized root vegetable related to carrots, although they don't really taste like carrots. Starchy with a mild sweet flavor, parsnips can be prepared in many ways as baby grows. They are a good source of vitamin C, folate, manganese, as well as complex carbohydrates (aka sustained energy) for your little one on the go. **MAKES ABOUT 1 CUP**

1 to 2 tablespoons coconut oil (optional)

3 parsnips, peeled and cut into ½-inch dice

¼ cup filtered water, plus more to thin to desired consistency

1 In a medium saucepan, heat the coconut oil over medium-low heat (if using). (Before making this recipe, you can introduce coconut oil by itself to test for any possible reaction.)

2 Add the parsnips and water. Cover with a lid, bring to a simmer, and cook for 5 to 8 minutes, or until very soft. Remove from the heat. Transfer to a blender. Purée, adding more water to thin to your desired consistency.

Storage: Keep in a glass jar in the refrigerator for up to 3 days.

Tip: If you're comfortable with dairy, you can use ghee or grass-fed butter instead of coconut oil. And for a non-vegetarian version, try using bone broth instead of water.

6 TO 8 MONTHS

All-Organic Baby Food Cookbook

Soft-Cooked Mushrooms

PREP TIME: 5 minutes **COOK TIME:** 10 minutes

FREEZER-FRIENDLY · BLW · **DAIRY-FREE** · **GLUTEN-FREE** · **NUT-FREE** · VEGAN · VEGETARIAN

I know, mushrooms aren't really a vegetable; they're a fungus! When your baby is closer to 8 months of age, mushrooms make an excellent soft-cooked finger food. Mushrooms have a high nutritional profile and antioxidant properties, which boost immunity and protect against disease. I recommend offering mushrooms regularly; they are so versatile, and in fact, they are one of the foods both my kids loved from a young age and still steal off my plate. SERVES ABOUT 4

2 to 3 tablespoons coconut oil

1 cup sliced baby portobello mushrooms, halved

1. In a small saucepan, heat the coconut oil over medium-high heat. (Before making this recipe, you can introduce coconut oil by itself to test for any possible reaction.)

2. Add the mushrooms. Cook, stirring occasionally, for 7 to 8 minutes, or until very soft and browned. Remove from the heat.

Storage: Keep in a glass jar in the refrigerator for up to 3 days or in an airtight glass container in the freezer for up to 6 months.

Tip: These mushrooms are really nice to add to a purée or serve alongside another soft-cooked finger food like zucchini. If you're comfortable with dairy, you can use ghee or grass-fed butter instead of coconut oil.

Soft-Cooked Summer Squash

PREP TIME: 10 minutes **COOK TIME:** 10 minutes
FREEZER-FRIENDLY · BLW · **DAIRY-FREE** · **GLUTEN-FREE** · **NUT-FREE** · **VEGAN** · **VEGETARIAN**

This peeled squash recipe is super-easy to offer as a soft-cooked finger food. Sometimes the peel gets in the way of new eaters at first, but once your baby has mastered this recipe, try cooking the squash with the peel on. Summer squash is related to green zucchini. They both have soft skin, which becomes even softer when cooked down. **MAKES ABOUT SIXTEEN 1-OUNCE FREEZER CUBES**

3 small yellow summer squash, peeled and diced

¼ cup filtered water

1 to 2 tablespoons coconut oil (optional)

1 In a medium saucepan, combine the squash, water, and coconut oil (if using). (Before making this recipe, you can introduce coconut oil by itself to test for any possible reaction.)

2 Cover with a lid, bring to a simmer over medium-low heat, and cook for 5 to 7 minutes, or until very soft. Remove from the heat.

Storage: Divide into ice cube trays, freeze overnight, and transfer to an airtight zip-top bag or glass container. Freeze for up to 6 months. You can alternatively save some in the refrigerator in a glass jar and divide the rest to freeze.

Tip: You can also transfer the cooked squash to a blender and purée, adding more water to reach your desired consistency. If you're comfortable with dairy, you can use ghee or grass-fed butter instead of coconut oil. And for a non-vegetarian version, try using bone broth instead of water.

Pairings: This recipe works with a dash of ground cumin or garlic powder.

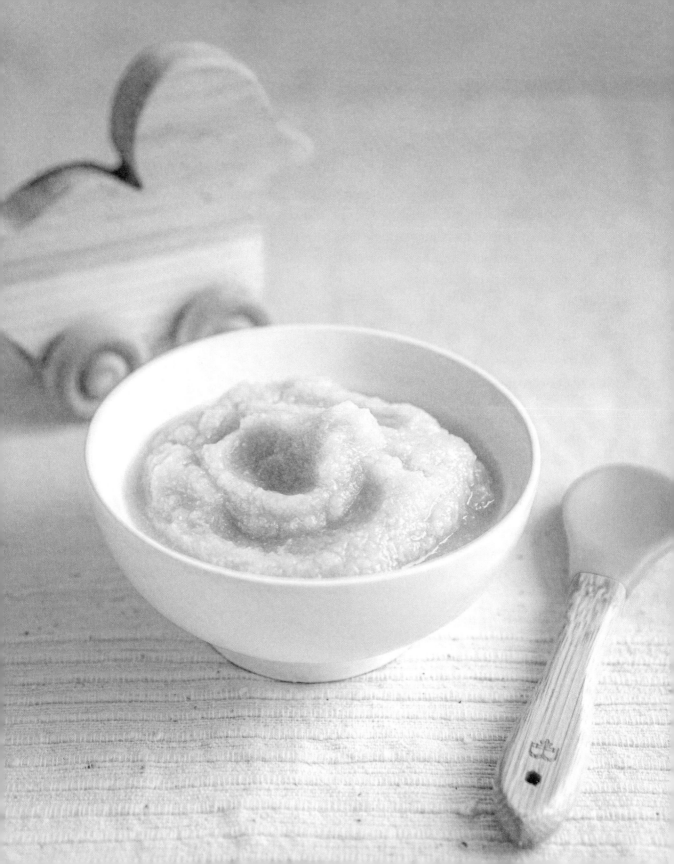

Asparagus Purée

PREP TIME: 5 minutes **COOK TIME:** 5 to 10 minutes

FREEZER-FRIENDLY · **DAIRY-FREE** · **GLUTEN-FREE** · **NUT-FREE** · **VEGAN** · **VEGETARIAN**

Asparagus contains a rich nutrient profile, including fat-soluble vitamins A, D, E, and K. This means you need a fat served with it to absorb these vitamins. Asparagus can be fun to offer your baby in a purée or as a cooked finger food. Asparagus can cause gas in some babies, much like cauliflower or broccoli, so if your baby is sensitive, it might be better to wait until closer to 9 or 10 months to introduce. Otherwise, this recipe is good for babies around 8 months. **MAKES ABOUT SIXTEEN 1-OUNCE FREEZER CUBES**

Filtered water

12 asparagus spears (about 1 ½ pounds), woody ends removed

1 to 2 tablespoons coconut oil (optional)

1   Set a steaming basket in a medium saucepan, and bring about 1 inch water to a boil, making sure the water does not touch the bottom of the basket.

2   Put the asparagus in the basket, tightly cover with a lid, and steam for 3 to 7 minutes, or until tender. Remove from the heat. Transfer to a blender.

3   Add the coconut oil (if using) and purée to your desired consistency. (Before making this recipe, you can introduce coconut oil by itself to test for any possible reaction.)

Storage: Divide into ice cube trays, freeze overnight, and transfer to an airtight zip-top bag or glass container. Freeze for up to 6 months. You can alternatively save some in a glass jar in the refrigerator for up to 3 days and divide the rest to freeze.

Tip: You can also serve as a finger food instead of puréeing. After cooking, just toss the asparagus in the oil before serving. If you're comfortable with dairy, you can use ghee or grass-fed butter instead of coconut oil.

Soft-Cooked Carrot Purée

PREP TIME: 10 minutes **COOK TIME:** 20 to 25 minutes
FREEZER-FRIENDLY · **DAIRY-FREE** · **GLUTEN-FREE** · **NUT-FREE** · **VEGAN** · **VEGETARIAN**

This particular recipe is so tasty, I find myself dipping a finger into the purée and eating it while I'm whipping it up for my babies. Packed with beta-carotene, which the body converts to vitamin A, carrots bring immunity-boosting properties and eye health to the table (literally and figuratively) for your little one. **MAKES ABOUT SIXTEEN 1-OUNCE FREEZER CUBES**

1 pound carrots, cut into 1-inch pieces

½ cup filtered water, plus more to thin to desired consistency

2 tablespoons coconut oil (optional)

1   In a pot, combine the carrots and water. Cook over medium heat for 20 to 25 minutes, or until very soft. Remove from the heat. Transfer to a blender.

2   Add the coconut oil (if using) and purée until smooth, creamy, and thick. (Before making this recipe, you can introduce coconut oil by itself to test for any possible reaction.) Add more water to reach your desired consistency.

Storage: Divide into ice cube trays, freeze overnight, and transfer to an airtight zip-top bag or glass container. Freeze for up to 6 months. You can alternatively save some in a glass jar in the refrigerator for up to 3 days and divide the rest to freeze.

Tip: If you're comfortable with dairy, you can use ghee or grass-fed butter instead of coconut oil. And for a non-vegetarian version, try using bone broth instead of water.

VEGGIE RECIPES

Soft-Cooked Broccoli

PREP TIME: 5 minutes **COOK TIME:** 10 to 15 minutes

FREEZER-FRIENDLY · **BLW** · **DAIRY-FREE** · **GLUTEN-FREE** · **NUT-FREE** · **VEGAN** · **VEGETARIAN**

Broccoli is rich in nutrients from the inside out. For growth and development, it contains iron and zinc, along with vitamins A, C, K, and B$_6$ and folate. As a cruciferous food, it can sometimes lead to gassiness, so waiting until your baby is at least 8 months of age is ideal. You can always test it out and see how your baby tolerates it, since every baby is different. Soft-cooked broccoli makes an excellent finger food. **MAKES ABOUT 2 CUPS**

Filtered water

1 head of broccoli, cut into florets

2 tablespoons extra-virgin olive oil or avocado oil

1 Set a steaming basket in a medium pot, and bring about 1 inch water to a boil, making sure the water does not touch the bottom of the basket.

2 Put the broccoli in the basket, tightly cover with a lid, and steam for 8 to 10 minutes, or until completely soft and the stems are easily pierced with a fork. Remove from the heat.

3 Cut each floret in half vertically, making sure to cut the round stalk, which can be a choking hazard. Transfer to a bowl.

4 Add the oil, and toss.

Storage: Keep in a glass jar in the refrigerator for up to 3 days or in an airtight glass storage container in the freezer for up to 3 months.

6 TO 8 MONTHS

All-Organic Baby Food Cookbook

Beet Mash or Purée

PREP TIME: 5 to 10 minutes **COOK TIME:** 10 to 15 minutes
FREEZER-FRIENDLY · **DAIRY-FREE** · **GLUTEN-FREE** · **NUT-FREE** · **VEGAN** · **VEGETARIAN**

This root veggie gets overlooked, but it's packed with beneficial fiber, potassium, folate, and more. Don't be alarmed: Your baby's poop will definitely have a red tinge to it after enjoying beets. Some sources recommend waiting until closer to 10 months of age for beets, but other sources say it's safe at 6 months of age or older. MAKES ABOUT 1 ½ CUPS

Filtered water

2 golden or red beets, peeled and cut into ½-inch dice

2 tablespoons coconut oil (optional)

1   Set a steaming basket in a medium pot, and bring about 1 inch water to a boil, making sure the water does not touch the bottom of the basket.

2   Put the beets in the basket, cover tightly with a lid, and steam for about 10 minutes, or until very tender. Remove from the heat. Transfer to a bowl, and mash with a fork.

3   If introducing around 6 to 7 months of age, transfer the beets to a blender instead, add the coconut oil (if using), and mash or purée. (Before making this recipe, you can introduce coconut oil by itself to test for any possible reaction.)

Storage: Keep in a glass jar in refrigerator for up to 3 days or in an airtight glass storage container in the freezer for up to 3 months.

Tip: If introducing this food to your baby around 8 months of age or older, cut into small, soft finger-food chunks, and serve with coconut oil. If you're comfortable with dairy, you can use ghee or grass-fed butter instead of coconut oil.

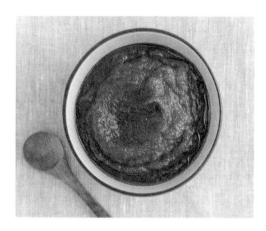

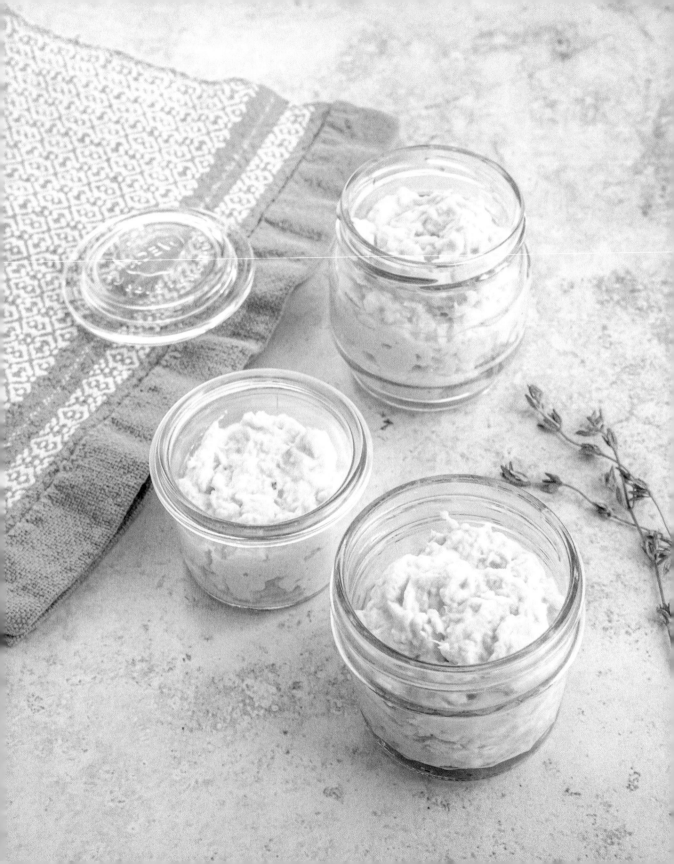

Chicken Purée

COOK TIME: 10 to 15 minutes

FREEZER-FRIENDLY · **DAIRY-FREE** · **GLUTEN-FREE** · **NUT-FREE**

Chicken is mild in flavor and pairs well with many vegetables or other foods your baby might already be eating. It's loaded with B complex vitamins (for energy), protein for growing babies, and iron. Around 9 to 10 months, you can offer a whole chicken drumstick to your baby for a more baby-led weaning approach. It's easy to hold, and safe for eating once you remove the skin, any loose bones, or pieces of loose fat. **MAKES ABOUT SIXTEEN 1-OUNCE FREEZER CUBES**

1 to 2 pounds boneless chicken breasts

3 to 4 cups filtered water

¼ teaspoon dried sage or thyme (optional)

In a pot, combine the chicken, water, and sage (if using). Cook over medium heat for 10 to 15 minutes, or until the chicken has cooked through. Remove from the heat. Transfer to a blender, and purée to your desired consistency.

Storage: Divide into ice cube trays, freeze overnight, and transfer to an airtight zip-top bag or glass container. Freeze for up to 6 months. You can alternatively save some in a glass jar in the refrigerator for up to 3 days and divide the rest to freeze.

Tip: You can try using bone broth instead of water. Instead of puréeing, you can cut the chicken into pea-size pieces and serve as is. Make sure the chicken is very tender.

Turkey Purée

COOK TIME: 10 to 15 minutes

FREEZER-FRIENDLY · **DAIRY-FREE** · **GLUTEN-FREE** · **NUT-FREE**

Turkey is another nutrient-rich meat that is mild in flavor and pairs well with many vegetables or other foods your baby might already be eating. It's loaded with B complex vitamins (for energy), protein for growing babies, and iron. The zinc and selenium found in turkey supports your baby's immune system. Ground turkey can be a great substitute for ground beef, while turkey can also sub in for chicken in many meals. **MAKES ABOUT SIXTEEN 1-OUNCE FREEZER CUBES**

1 to 2 pounds boneless turkey breasts

3 to 4 cups filtered water

¼ teaspoon dried sage or thyme (optional)

In a pot, combine the turkey, water, and sage (if using). Cook over medium heat for 10 to 15 minutes, or until the turkey has cooked through. Remove from the heat. Transfer to a blender and purée to your desired consistency.

Storage: Divide into ice cube trays, freeze overnight, and transfer to an airtight zip-top bag or glass container. Freeze for up to 6 months. You can alternatively save some in a glass jar in the refrigerator for up to 3 days and divide the rest to freeze.

Tip: You can try using bone broth instead of water, and if breasts are unavailable, you can use ground turkey. Instead of puréeing, you can cut the turkey into pea-size pieces and serve as is.

Pork Purée

COOK TIME: 10 minutes

FREEZER-FRIENDLY · DAIRY-FREE · GLUTEN-FREE · NUT-FREE

Pork isn't one of the first things you might think of to feed a baby, maybe because a lot of pork comes in the form of sausage or other preserved varieties that are high in sodium. The sodium content in those types of pork are too much for a baby's small kidneys. Ground pork, however, from a pasture-raised, nitrate-free source, can be really beneficial for your baby. It's high in protein, selenium for a happy thyroid that equals healthy hormone production, and B vitamins. Some babies are ready around 8 months of age for ground pork, either as a finger food or mixed into an already introduced vegetable purée. However, others may do best with it puréed at this age.

MAKES 1 TO 1 ½ CUPS

1 pound pasture-raised ground pork

¼ cup filtered water

1 Heat a medium skillet over medium heat.

2 Add the pork and cook, breaking up the meat, for 7 to 8 minutes, or until no longer pink. Remove from the heat. Drain and discard the fat.

3 Transfer the pork to a blender, and purée to your desired consistency, adding the water as needed.

Storage: Keep in a glass jar in the refrigerator for up to 3 days.

Tip: Instead of puréeing, you can break up the pork into pea-size pieces and serve as is.

Pairings: You can also serve the pork mixed with bone broth, a puréed vegetable such as sweet potatoes or carrots, or full-fat, plain yogurt, if it has already been introduced.

Beef Purée

COOK TIME: 10 minutes

FREEZER-FRIENDLY · **DAIRY-FREE** · **GLUTEN-FREE** · **NUT-FREE**

Beef is one of the best iron sources for your baby. If you aren't introducing any of the Superfoods for Babies (page 49), like liver pâté or bone marrow, pasture-raised or grass-fed beef is going to be your next-best animal source for iron. It's high in protein, iron, and B vitamins. Some babies are ready around 8 months of age for ground beef, either as a finger food or mixed into an already introduced vegetable purée. However, others may do best with it puréed at this age. **MAKES 1 TO 1 ½ CUPS**

1 pound grass-fed ground beef

¼ cup filtered water

1   Heat a medium skillet over medium heat.

2   Add the beef and cook, breaking up the meat, for 8 to 10 minutes, or until no longer pink. Remove from the heat. Drain and discard the fat.

3   Transfer the beef to a blender, and purée to your desired consistency, adding the water as needed.

Storage: Keep in a glass jar in the refrigerator for up to 3 days.

Tip: Bison is a really great alternative here. They are not mass produced like beef cattle. Instead of puréeing, you can break up the beef into pea-size pieces and serve as is.

Pairings: You can also serve the beef mixed with bone broth, a puréed vegetable such as sweet potatoes, butternut squash, or zucchini, or full-fat, plain yogurt, if it has already been introduced.

Lamb Purée

COOK TIME: 5 to 10 minutes

FREEZER-FRIENDLY · **DAIRY-FREE** · **GLUTEN-FREE** · **NUT-FREE**

Lamb is another meat you probably wouldn't think to serve your baby right off the bat, but it's an exceptional source of heme iron, B vitamins, zinc, and selenium for hormone health. Some babies around 8 months of age are ready for ground lamb, either as a finger food or mixed into an already intro-duced vegetable purée. However, others may do best with it puréed at this age. **MAKES 1 TO 1 ½ CUPS**

1 pound ground lamb

Filtered water

1   Heat a medium skillet over medium-high heat.

2   Add the lamb and cook, breaking up the meat, for 5 to 6 minutes, or until no longer pink. Remove from the heat. Drain and discard the fat.

3   Transfer the lamb to a blender, and purée to your desired consistency, adding the water as needed.

Storage: Keep in a glass jar in the refrig-erator for up to 3 days.

Tip: Instead of puréeing, you can break up the lamb into pea-size pieces and serve as is.

Pairings: You can also serve the lamb mixed with bone broth, a puréed veg-etable such as sweet potatoes, butternut squash, or zucchini, or full-fat, plain yogurt, if it has already been introduced.

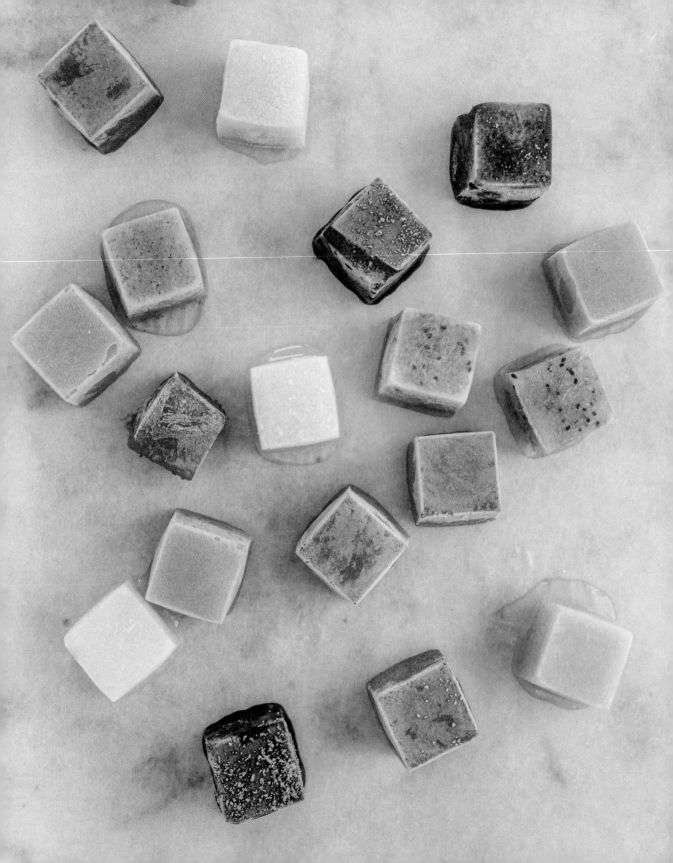

Six

Adventurous Flavors

7 TO 8 MONTHS

The recipes in this chapter are more adventurous in texture and flavor, keeping things exciting and helping to develop your baby's broad palate. Just think, your hard work will pay off when your baby grows into a toddler and isn't scared to try new foods! The recipes in this chapter include the introduction of fish and combination purées of fruits and veggies. Your baby might give you a funny face with new textures, but it's important to keep offering them so baby can get used to it. Don't let any long-standing bias you may have against food stop you. You are doing your little one a great service by offering lots of variety of foods, flavors, and textures. And who knows, their response might inspire you to try them again!

WHAT TO EXPECT

For now, baby's main source of nutrition will remain breast milk or formula. Variety in texture and flavor is what's desired here. Foods should be thicker than they have been so far and include some very soft, mushy lumps, easily mashable with their hard gums (even if they have no teeth).

How Much to Feed
2 tablespoons to ¼ cup, following baby's lead

When to Feed
About twice a day. A sample pattern would be: wake up, nurse/bottle, mid-morning meal (introduce a new food), nurse/bottle before an afternoon nap, dinner with the family (already-introduced food), and nurse/bottle before bed.

What to Drink
About one ounce of water or bone broth in a sippy cup or open cup (starting at 6 months old). This will allow them to wash food down and learn to drink from a cup.

First-Time Parent Tip

The more babies get to experience a range of textures and flavors at an early age, the more likely they will be to continue to enjoy different foods as they grow. In other words, you're essentially laying the foundation for an adventurous eater. Every parent wants this in the end, and it starts with what we offer in the beginning months and years.

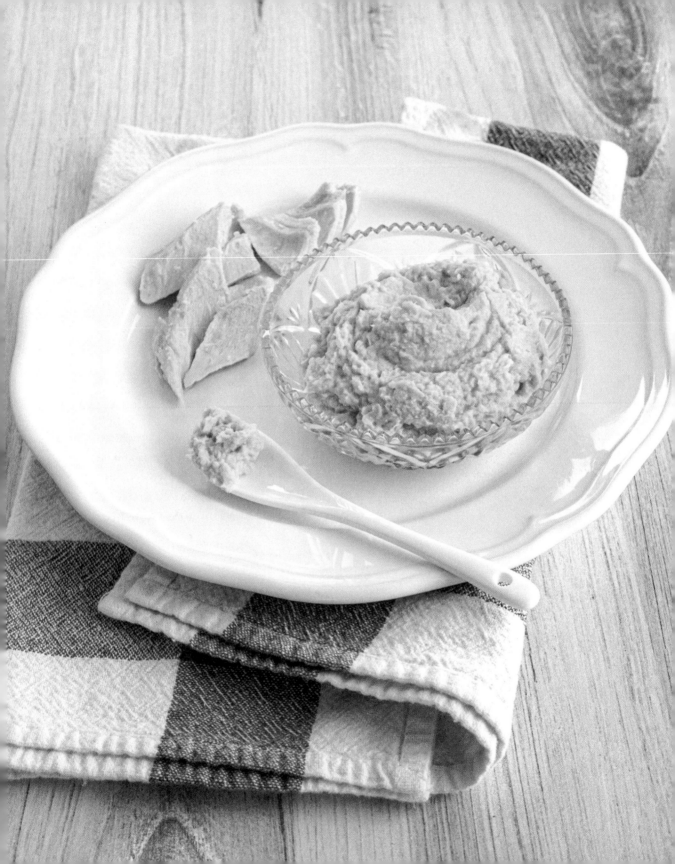

Salmon Purée

PREP TIME: 10 minutes **COOK TIME:** 10 to 15 minutes
FREEZER-FRIENDLY · **DAIRY-FREE** · **GLUTEN-FREE** · **NUT-FREE**

Salmon is wonderfully rich in omega-3s and fatty acids (DHA and EPA) for brain, nerve, and eye development. Experts used to recommend holding off on fish until your baby is bigger, but it's since been proven that introducing it around this age offers better protection against fish allergies. Kids also tend to develop strong preferences for food before age 5, so make sure to introduce fish often. That way, they'll acquire that good love and taste for healthy seafood early on. **MAKES ABOUT ¾ CUP**

1 to 2 cups filtered water, plus more to thin to desired consistency

2 tablespoons coconut oil

2 (4- to 6-ounce) wild-caught salmon fillets, pin bones removed

1 In a medium saucepan, bring the water and coconut oil to a simmer over medium-low heat. (Before making this recipe, you can introduce coconut oil by itself to test for any possible reaction.)

2 Add the salmon, making sure it's immersed. Cover with a lid, and cook for 6 to 10 minutes, or until the flesh flakes easily with a fork and has cooked through. Remove from the heat. Transfer to a blender, and purée to your desired consistency, adding water as needed.

Storage: Divide into ice cube trays, freeze overnight, and transfer to an airtight zip-top bag or glass container. Freeze for up to 6 months. You can alternatively save some in a glass jar in the refrigerator for up to 3 days and divide the rest to freeze.

Tip: You can try using bone broth instead of water, and if you're comfortable with dairy, you can use ghee or grass-fed butter instead of coconut oil. Instead of puréeing, you can break the fish into small pieces and serve as is.

Trout Purée

PREP TIME: 5 minutes **COOK TIME:** 10 to 15 minutes

FREEZER-FRIENDLY · **DAIRY-FREE** · **GLUTEN-FREE** · **NUT-FREE**

Trout contains selenium, which combined with vitamin E, acts as an antioxidant. Selenium helps immune function and supports the body's ability to detox. It's also rich in omega-3s and fatty acids (DHA and EPA) for brain, nerve, and eye development. It's been proven that introducing fish around this age is better protection against fish allergies. Another good reason not to wait is that kids tend to develop strong preferences for food before age 5. Introducing fish often will help them acquire a taste for healthy seafood early on. **MAKES ABOUT ¾ CUP**

1 to 2 cups filtered water, plus more to thin to desired consistency

2 tablespoons coconut oil

1 teaspoon grated lemon zest

2 (4- to 6-ounce) trout fillets

1   In a medium saucepan, combine the water, coconut oil, and lemon zest. Bring to a simmer over medium-low heat. (Before making this recipe, you can introduce coconut oil by itself to test for any possible reaction).

2   Add the trout, making sure it's immersed. Cover with a lid, and cook for 6 to 10 minutes, or until the flesh flakes easily with a fork and has cooked through. Remove from the heat. Transfer to a blender, and purée to your desired consistency, adding water as needed.

Storage: Divide into ice cube trays, freeze overnight, and transfer to an airtight zip-top bag or glass container. Freeze for up to 6 months. You can alternatively save some in a glass jar in the refrigerator for up to 3 days and divide the rest to freeze.

Tip: You can try using bone broth instead of water, and if you're comfortable with dairy, you can use ghee or grass-fed butter instead of coconut oil. Instead of puréeing, you can break the fish into small pieces and serve as is.

Cod Purée

PREP TIME: 5 minutes **COOK TIME:** 10 to 15 minutes
FREEZER-FRIENDLY · **DAIRY-FREE** · **GLUTEN-FREE** · **NUT-FREE**

Cod is rich in B complexes, vitamins C and E, potassium, and magnesium. Like other fish, cod is rich in omega-3s and fatty acids (DHA and EPA) for brain, nerve, and eye development. Current research shows that introducing fish around this age offers better protection against fish allergies. Since kids tend to develop strong preferences for food before age 5, you'll want to introduce fish often so they acquire a taste for healthy seafood at a young age. **MAKES ABOUT ¾ CUP**

1 to 2 cups filtered water

2 tablespoons coconut oil

1 teaspoon grated lemon zest

2 (4- to 6-ounce) cod fillets

1   In a medium saucepan, combine the water, coconut oil, and lemon zest. Bring to a simmer over medium-low heat. (Before making this recipe, you can introduce coconut oil by itself to test for any possible reaction.)

2   Add the cod, making sure it's immersed. Cover with a lid, and cook for 6 to 10 minutes, or until the flesh flakes easily with a fork and has cooked through. Remove from the heat. Transfer to a blender, and purée to your desired consistency, adding water as needed.

Storage: Divide into ice cube trays, freeze overnight, then transfer to an airtight zip-top bag or glass container. Freeze for up to 6 months. You can alternatively save some in a glass jar in the refrigerator for up to 3 days and divide the rest to freeze.

Tip: You can try using bone broth instead of water, and if you're comfortable with dairy, you can use ghee or grass-fed butter instead of coconut oil. Instead of puréeing, you can break the fish into small pieces and serve as is.

Salmon and Mango Purée

PREP TIME: 10 minutes **COOK TIME:** 10 minutes
FREEZER-FRIENDLY · **DAIRY-FREE** · **GLUTEN-FREE** · **NUT-FREE**

Salmon and all its goodness (healthy omegas and fats) pairs really well with mango. Whether you purée this dish or serve it as finger food, it's a winning combination and pretty to look at. For added nutrition, texture, and color, I like to serve it alongside an Avocado Mash (page 65). **MAKES ABOUT 1 ½ CUPS**

2 ½ cups filtered water

¼ pound wild-caught salmon fillets, pin bones removed

1 cup frozen mango chunks

1 Set a steaming basket in a large pot, and bring 2 cups of water to a boil, making sure the water does not touch the bottom of the basket.

2 Place the salmon, skin-side down, and mango in the basket. Reduce the heat to a simmer, tightly cover with a lid, and steam for about 8 minutes, or until the salmon flakes easily with a fork and has cooked through. Remove from the heat. Let cool with the lid off. Transfer to a blender.

3 Add the remaining ½ cup of water, and purée until smooth.

Storage: Keep in a glass jar in the refrigerator for up to 3 days. Or divide into ice cube trays, freeze overnight, and transfer to an airtight zip-top bag or glass container. Freeze for up to 6 months.

Tip: You can try using bone broth instead of water. And instead of puréeing, you can serve as finger foods to your baby alongside mashed (or even sliced) avocado.

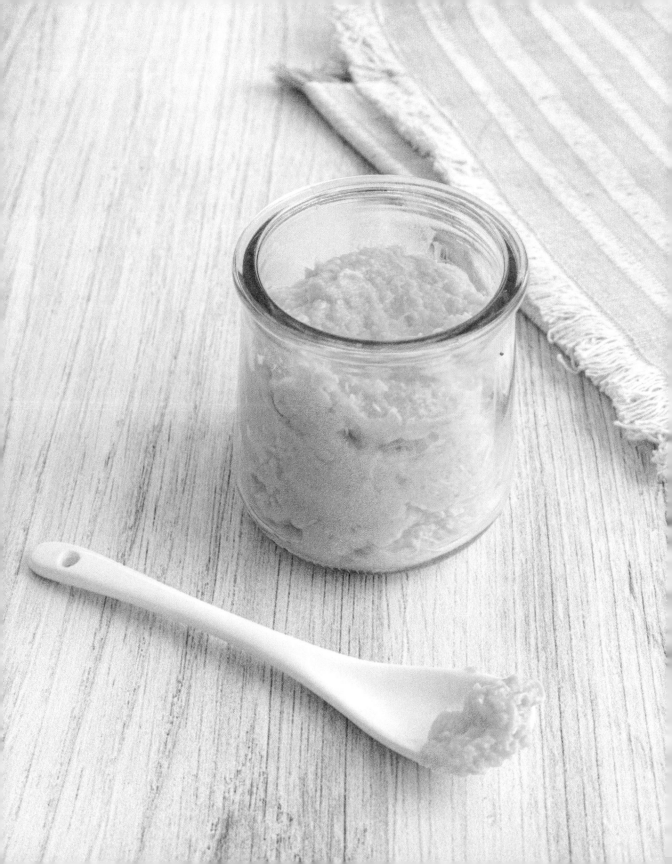

Sardine Rillette Mash

PREP TIME: 5 minutes

FREEZER-FRIENDLY · **DAIRY-FREE OPTION** · **GLUTEN-FREE** · **NUT-FREE**

I was unintentionally making this common French appetizer for my son Aldrik with other canned fish like mackerel when he started solids. It wasn't until recently that I found out sardines make a perfect rillette, or meat spread. Sardines are a low-mercury fish and high in calcium, making them top choices for babies. They are a close second to salmon for omega-3 fatty acid and DHA content, which both fuel eye, brain, and immunity development. Because sardines come in a can, make sure they are labeled BPA-free and choose a low-sodium variety. **MAKES ABOUT ¾ CUP**

1 (4-ounce) can low-sodium sardines in olive oil, drained and rinsed

2 to 3 tablespoons full-fat, plain yogurt or avocado oil–based mayonnaise

1 tablespoon olive oil

1 teaspoon fresh parsley leaves, minced

1 teaspoon fresh lemon juice (optional)

In a small bowl, combine the sardines, yogurt, olive oil, parsley, and lemon juice (if using). Using a spoon or fork, mash.

Storage: Store a glass jar in the refrigerator for up to 2 to 3 days.

Tip: The bones in sardines are tiny, soft, and crushable with a spoon or fork. Alternatively, you could make this with anchovies, or use avocado or extra olive oil in place of the yogurt for a dairy-free version.

Shrimp and Plantain Purée

PREP TIME: 10 minutes **COOK TIME:** 10 minutes
FREEZER-FRIENDLY · **DAIRY-FREE** · **GLUTEN-FREE** · **NUT-FREE**

Plantains look like bananas, but they aren't as sweet and are typically not eaten raw. They make a delicious starchy cooked fruit. This shrimp and plantain combo makes for a perfect southern combination for your baby, while introducing the common allergen shellfish. **MAKES ABOUT SIXTEEN 1-OUNCE FREEZER CUBES**

1 tablespoon coconut oil

1 green plantain, peeled and sliced

1 cup frozen shrimp, thawed

2 teaspoons tomato paste

1 cup filtered water

1 In a medium saucepan, heat the coconut oil over medium heat.

2 Add the plantain and cook for 3 minutes, then flip.

3 Add the shrimp. Cook for 2 minutes, flip, and cook for 1 minute.

4 Add the tomato paste and water, stirring to combine. Bring to a boil. Remove from the heat. Transfer to a blender, and purée to your desired consistency.

Storage: Divide into ice cube trays, freeze overnight, and transfer to an airtight zip-top bag or glass container. Freeze for up to 6 months. You can alternatively save some in a glass jar in the refrigerator for up to 3 days and divide the rest to freeze.

Tip: You can try using bone broth instead of water, and if you're comfortable with dairy, you can use ghee instead of coconut oil.

Chicken and Carrot Purée

PREP TIME: 5 minutes **COOK TIME:** 10 to 15 minutes
FREEZER-FRIENDLY · **DAIRY-FREE** · **GLUTEN-FREE** · **NUT-FREE**

With its mild flavor, chicken pairs well with many vegetables or other foods your baby might already be eating. It's loaded with B complex vitamins (for energy), protein vital for growing babies, and iron. Adding some carrot here gives the warm, cozy taste of a chicken noodle soup (just save the noodles until your baby is a bit older). **MAKES ABOUT SIXTEEN 1-OUNCE FREEZER CUBES**

1 boneless, skinless chicken breast

1 carrot, chopped

¾ to 1 cup filtered water

¼ teaspoon dried sage or thyme (optional)

Tip: You can try using bone broth instead of water. Instead of puréeing, you can break up the chicken into pea-size pieces and serve as is.

1   In a pot, combine the chicken, carrot, water, and sage (if using). Cover with a lid, and cook over medium heat for 10 to 15 minutes, or until the chicken has cooked through and the carrot is soft.

2   Remove from the heat. Transfer to a blender, and purée to your desired consistency.

Storage: Divide into ice cube trays, freeze overnight, and transfer to an airtight zip-top bag or glass container. Freeze for up to 6 months. You can alternatively save some in a glass jar in the refrigerator for up to 3 days and divide the rest to freeze.

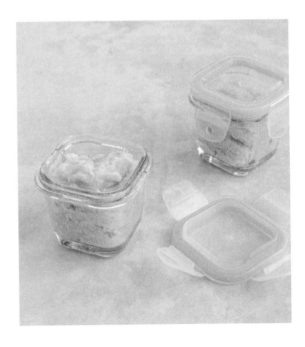

Chicken and Avocado Purée

PREP TIME: 5 minutes **COOK TIME:** 10 to 15 minutes
FREEZER-FRIENDLY · **DAIRY-FREE** · **GLUTEN-FREE** · **NUT-FREE**

Chicken is a versatile meat that can be combined with many of the vegetables or other foods your baby might already be eating. In this purée, we'll combine chicken with some creamy avocado for a tasty superfood combo full of healthy fats, fiber, B vitamins, as well as vitamins C, E, and K, protein, and iron—to name just a few! **MAKES ABOUT SIXTEEN 1-OUNCE FREEZER CUBES**

1 boneless, skinless chicken breast

1 ripe avocado, pitted, peeled, and sliced

¾ to 1 cup filtered water

¼ teaspoon dried sage or thyme (optional)

1 In a pot, combine the chicken, avocado, water, and sage (if using). Cover with a lid, and cook over medium heat for 10 to 15 minutes, or until the chicken has cooked through.

2 Remove from the heat. Transfer to a blender, and purée to your desired consistency.

Storage: Divide into ice cube trays, freeze overnight, then transfer to an airtight zip-top bag or glass container. Freeze for up to 6 months. You can alternatively save some in a glass jar in the refrigerator for up to 3 days and divide the rest to freeze.

Tip: You can try using bone broth instead of water. Instead of puréeing, you can break up the chicken into pea-size pieces and serve alongside avocado.

Ground Beef with Butternut Squash Mash

PREP TIME: 10 minutes **COOK TIME:** 30 to 45 minutes

FREEZER-FRIENDLY · **DAIRY-FREE** · **GLUTEN-FREE** · **NUT-FREE**

Squash is packed with vitamin C, fiber, and beta-carotene (vitamin A). Beta-carotene is incredible for our body's health, associated with a reduced risk of cancer, diabetes, heart and respiratory diseases, and more. Serving squash with the heme-iron-rich beef makes for a powerful combo for babies, and the flavor is pretty great, too. **MAKES ABOUT 5 CUPS**

1 small butternut squash, halved lengthwise and seeded

4 tablespoons avocado oil

1 tablespoon minced garlic

1 pound grass-fed ground beef

1 Preheat the oven to 400°F. Line a baking sheet with parchment paper.

2 Drizzle the cut sides of the squash with 2 tablespoons of avocado oil, and place, cut-side down, on the prepared baking sheet.

3 Transfer the baking sheet to the oven, and bake for 30 to 45 minutes, or until the squash is soft and the skin is starting to get wrinkly. Remove from the oven.

4 Meanwhile, in a skillet, heat the remaining 2 tablespoons of avocado oil over medium heat.

5 Add the garlic and cook for 1 minute.

6 Add the beef. Cook, breaking up the meat, for 8 to 10 minutes, or until no longer pink. Remove from the heat.

7 Scrape out the flesh from the squash, transfer to a bowl, and discard the shell. Mash the beef mixture into it.

Storage: Keep in an airtight glass container in the refrigerator for up to 3 days or freeze leftovers for up to 6 months..

Tip: You can try using bone broth instead of water.

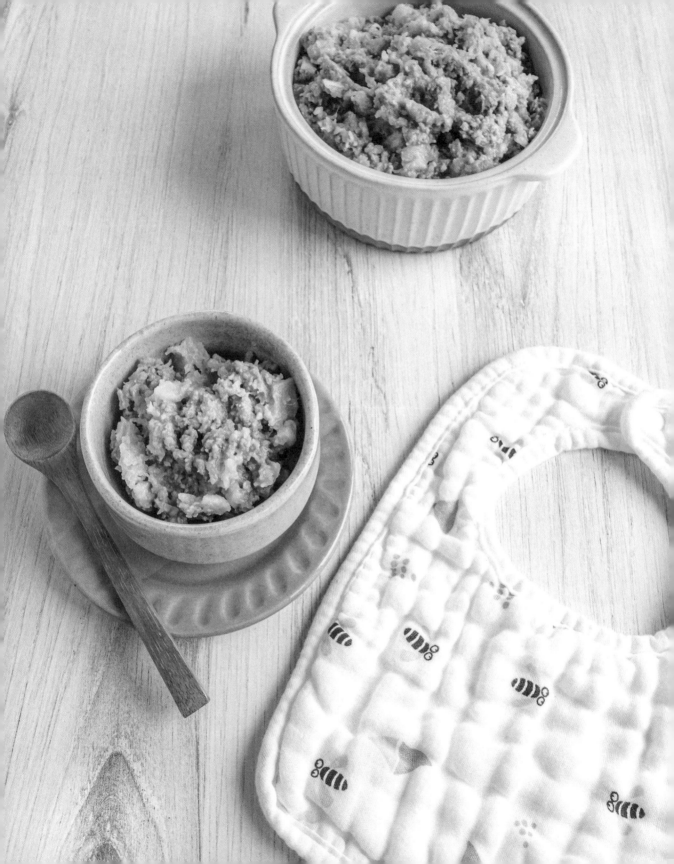

Berries with Coconut Cream

PREP TIME: 5 minutes, plus a few hours to chill the coconut milk
COOK TIME: 5 to 10 minutes
DAIRY-FREE · **GLUTEN-FREE** · **NUT-FREE** · **VEGAN** · **VEGETARIAN**

Raw berries can be rough on digestion for some babies, so cooking them
is best for a few more months. You can certainly try raw berries, but this
favorite breakfast treat with cooked berries is more easily digestible, which
provides optimal nutrient absorption. Berries are rich in antioxidants and
anti-inflammatory compounds. Coconut cream is high in lauric acid, meaning it contains antibacterial, antifungal, and antiviral properties, similar to
the magic of breast milk. Cold, canned coconut cream is a perfect vehicle for
babies to practice self-feeding, because it scoops easily without sliding off the
spoon. **MAKES ABOUT 3 CUPS**

1 tablespoon coconut oil

½ cup strawberries, hulled and sliced

½ cup blueberries

1 (15-ounce) can full-fat coconut milk, chilled

1   In a saucepan, heat the coconut oil over
    medium heat.

2   Add the strawberries and blueber-
    ries. Cook, mashing and stirring, for
    5 to 10 minutes, or until soft and warm.
    Remove from the heat.

3   Reserving the liquid for another use,
    scoop ¼ cup of cream (settled on
    the top) from the coconut milk into a
    bowl. Serve it topped with a scoop of
    mashed fruit.

Storage: Store leftover fruit and coconut
cream in separate airtight glass containers
in the refrigerator for up to 2 to 3 days.

Tip: You could also use another warmed
fruit, like peaches, apples, or pears. If
you're comfortable with dairy, you can use
ghee instead of coconut oil.

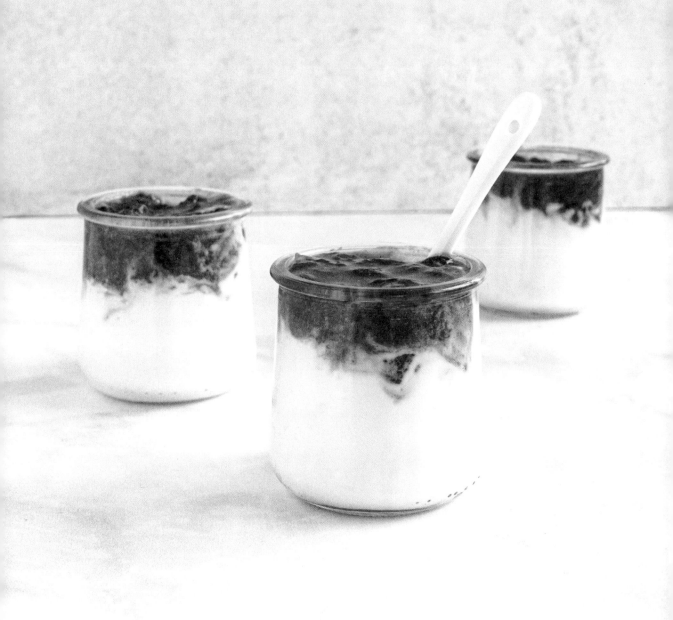

Soft-Cooked Beef, Parsnips, and Mushrooms

PREP TIME: 15 minutes **COOK TIME:** 15 to 20 minutes

FREEZER-FRIENDLY · **DAIRY-FREE** · **GLUTEN-FREE** · **NUT-FREE**

Once you've served these foods individually, this soft-cooked recipe is best served around 8 months of age or older as finger foods. The soft-cooked veggies and beef offer your baby wonderful opportunities to practice the pincer grasp. Introducing basil here brings a little oomph of flavor to this savory dish. **MAKES ABOUT 3 ½ CUPS**

2 tablespoons olive oil

1 pound grass-fed ground beef

½ onion, diced

1 to 2 teaspoons minced garlic

1 ½ cups diced (1-inch) parsnips

1 ½ cups mushrooms, diced

1 tablespoon fresh basil, finely chopped or 1 teaspoon dried

1 cup filtered water

1 Heat a medium skillet over medium heat. Add the olive oil.

2 Add the beef and cook, breaking up the meat, for 8 to 10 minutes, or until no longer pink. Transfer to a plate.

3 In the same skillet, add the onion and garlic. Cook for about 2 minutes, or until fragrant.

4 Add the parsnips, mushrooms, basil, and water. Stir, and bring to a simmer. Cover with a lid, and cook for 5 to 7 minutes, or until very tender.

5 Return the beef to the skillet, and stir to combine. Remove from the heat.

Storage: Keep in an airtight glass container in the refrigerator for up to 3 days or freeze leftovers for up to 6 months..

Tip: You could use carrots instead of parsnips and beef bone broth instead of water. You can also turn this into a mash by transferring the parsnips to a bowl, mashing them, then stirring in a bit of the beef and mushrooms.

Roasted Beet and Sweet Potato Mash

PREP TIME: 5 minutes **COOK TIME:** 45 minutes
FREEZER-FRIENDLY · **DAIRY-FREE** · **GLUTEN-FREE** · **NUT-FREE** · **VEGAN** · **VEGETARIAN**

This mash, packed with fiber, potassium, vitamin C, and more, is savory and sweet, satiating, and flavorful. The combination of the root vegetables is sure to captivate your baby's eye with the beautiful rich colors. Don't be alarmed: Your baby's poop will definitely have a red tinge to it from the beets!

MAKES ABOUT SIXTEEN 1-OUNCE FREEZER CUBES

1 sweet potato, halved lengthwise

1 golden or red beet, halved lengthwise

2 tablespoons coconut oil

1   Preheat the oven to 425°F. Line a baking sheet with parchment paper.

2   Place the sweet potato and beet halves, cut-side down, on the prepared baking sheet.

3   Transfer the baking sheet to the oven, and roast for about 45 minutes, or until cooked through. Remove from the oven. Let cool, then peel. Transfer to a bowl.

4   Add the coconut oil and mash.

Storage: Divide into ice cube trays, freeze overnight, and transfer to an airtight zip-top bag or glass container. Freeze for up to 6 months. You can alternatively save some in a glass jar in the refrigerator for up to 3 days and divide the rest to freeze.

Tip: If you're comfortable with dairy, you can use ghee or grass-fed butter instead of coconut oil.

Pumpkin and Apple Purée

PREP TIME: 15 to 20 minutes **COOK TIME:** 20 to 25 minutes
FREEZER-FRIENDLY · DAIRY-FREE · GLUTEN-FREE · NUT-FREE · VEGAN · VEGETARIAN

Capitalize on the season with this combination of apples and pumpkins, two fall favorites. Pie pumpkins (smaller than carving pumpkins) are most available in fall through early winter, and will last quite a while if stored in a cool, dark, dry place. If you can't find fresh pumpkin, frozen pumpkin, already nicely seeded and chopped, is a fine substitute. Packed with vitamins A and C, pumpkins are good for your little one's eyes and immune system. **MAKES ABOUT SIXTEEN 1-OUNCE FREEZER CUBES**

2 tablespoons coconut oil

1 pound pumpkin, peeled, seeded, and cut into ½-inch dice (about 1 ½ cups)

Filtered water

1 pound apples (about 3 apples), cored and cut into 1-inch dice

½ teaspoon ground cinnamon

1   In a medium pot, heat the coconut oil over low heat.

2   Add the pumpkin and cover with about ½ inch water. Cover with a lid, bring to a simmer, and cook for 5 minutes.

3   Add the apples, replace the lid, and simmer for 10 to 15 minutes, or until the pumpkin and apples are very soft. Remove from the heat. Transfer to a blender.

4   Add the cinnamon and purée to your desired consistency, adding water as needed.

Storage: Divide into ice cube trays, freeze overnight, and transfer to an airtight zip-top bag or glass container. Freeze for up to 6 months. You can alternatively save some in a glass jar in the refrigerator for up to 3 days and divide the rest to freeze.

Tip: Always wash pumpkins before cutting them, since they grow on the ground and can contain bacteria. If you're comfortable with dairy, you can use ghee instead of coconut oil.

Curry Cauliflower and Carrot Purée

PREP TIME: 5 to 10 minutes **COOK TIME:** 20 minutes
FREEZER-FRIENDLY · **DAIRY-FREE** · **GLUTEN-FREE** · **NUT-FREE** · **VEGAN** · **VEGETARIAN**

Yellow curry is safe for babies around 8 months of age. Curry powder is actually a combination of warming, yellow spices, primarily ginger and turmeric. These spices aid digestion and wellness for your little one while exposing them to broad flavors. Cauliflower is a cruciferous food, which has sulfur-containing compounds called glucosinolates, which may help prevent cancer. **MAKES ABOUT SIXTEEN 1-OUNCE FREEZER CUBES**

Filtered water

3 carrots, cut into ½-inch-thick pieces

1 cup cauliflower florets

¼ to ¾ teaspoon yellow curry powder

2 tablespoons coconut oil

1 Set a steaming basket in a medium sauce-pan, and bring 2 inches water to a boil, making sure the water does not touch the bottom of the basket.

2 Put the carrots in the basket, tightly cover with a lid, and steam for about 5 minutes, or until tender.

3 Add the cauliflower and replace the lid. Steam for about 10 minutes, or until the cauliflower is also tender. Remove from the heat. Transfer to a blender.

4 Add the curry powder and coconut oil. Purée to your desired consistency, adding water as needed.

Storage: Divide into ice cube trays, freeze overnight, and transfer to an airtight zip-top bag or glass container. Freeze for up to 6 months. You can alternatively save some in a glass jar in the refrigerator for up to 3 days and divide the rest to freeze.

Tip: You could use ground ginger, turmeric, or ground cumin instead of yellow curry, but stick with ⅛ teaspoon if you use ginger. If you're comfortable with dairy, you can use ghee instead of coconut oil. And for a non-vegetarian version, try using bone broth instead of water. This recipe makes for a nice finger food option, too.

Spiced Pear and Prune Purée

PREP TIME: 10 minutes **COOK TIME:** 15 minutes
FREEZER-FRIENDLY · **DAIRY-FREE** · **GLUTEN-FREE** · **NUT-FREE** · **VEGAN** · **VEGETARIAN**

Prunes may not be a part of your typical diet, but for babies, they can be a useful mainstay! This nutrient-dense combo is sure to get your baby's bowels moving if they're constipated. Pears and prunes alone will do this, but combining them with cloves makes it a warming blend for digestion. See the tip for alternate spice combinations. **MAKES TEN 1-OUNCE FREEZER CUBES**

¼ cup filtered water, plus more for cooking

2 ripe pears, cored and chopped

4 dried prunes, pitted

1 cup hot filtered water

⅛ teaspoon ground cloves

1 ½ tablespoons coconut oil

1 Set a steaming basket in a small saucepan, add 2 inches water, and bring to a boil, making sure the water does not touch the bottom of the basket.

2 Put the pears in the basket, tightly cover with a lid, and steam for about 10 minutes, or until soft. Remove from the heat. Transfer to a blender.

3 Meanwhile, in a small bowl, combine the prunes and hot water. Soak for 10 minutes, and drain.

4 Add the prunes, cloves, and coconut oil to the blender. Purée until smooth, adding water as needed. Strain through a fine-mesh sieve. Serve warm to aid with digestion and constipation.

Storage: Divide into ice cube trays, freeze overnight, and transfer to an airtight zip-top bag or glass container. Freeze for up to 6 months. You can alternatively save some in a glass jar in the refrigerator for up to 3 days and divide the rest to freeze.

Tip: Alternatively, you could use ⅛ teaspoon ground cinnamon or nutmeg instead of cloves.

Coconut Cream and Peach Purée

PREP TIME: 5 minutes, plus a few hours to chill the coconut milk
COOK TIME: 15 to 20 minutes
DAIRY-FREE · **GLUTEN-FREE** · **NUT-FREE** · **VEGAN** · **VEGETARIAN**

Coconut cream is high in lauric acid, which has antibacterial, antifungal, and antiviral effects. That means it can kill fungi, viruses, and bacteria, much like breast milk. Cold, canned coconut cream is a perfect way for babies to practice self-feeding because it scoops easily without sliding off the spoon. The peaches add color, flavor, and texture, a trifecta of variables your baby will love. Once these ingredients have been introduced separately, you can make this delicious antioxidant meal for your baby. **MAKES ABOUT 3 ½ CUPS**

2 tablespoons coconut oil

1 cup chopped peeled ripe peaches

1 (15-ounce) can full-fat coconut milk, chilled

1 In a pot, heat the coconut oil over medium-high heat.

2 Add the peaches and cook for 10 to 15 minutes, or until very soft. Remove from the heat. Let cool for a few minutes. Transfer to a blender, and purée until smooth, adding a splash of filtered water as needed.

3 Reserving the liquid for another use, scoop a quarter or half of the cream from the coconut milk into a bowl.

4 Mix in the warm peach purée.

Storage: Store the rest of the cream in a glass jar in the refrigerator, covered, for 1 to 2 days. It can also be served on its own, mixed with meats, or used as a dairy substitute in soups.

Tip: Allow your baby to self-feed with a preloaded spoon, or gently guide them to scoop and feed themselves.

Pairings: I love to serve coconut cream with fruits that have been introduced up to this point. Mango or berries pair well. For babies over 12 months of age, a drizzle of maple syrup or honey makes a special treat.

Root Veggie Purée

PREP TIME: 10 to 15 minutes **COOK TIME:** 30 minutes
FREEZER-FRIENDLY · DAIRY-FREE · GLUTEN-FREE · NUT-FREE · VEGAN · VEGETARIAN

This smooth root vegetable purée provides important nutrients and a new combination of flavors for your baby. Parsnips are related to parsley and carrots. Creamy in color, parsnips have a mildly sweet flavor that increases after a winter frost. By introducing thyme along with the vegetables, your baby will experience a tasty new combination. **MAKES ABOUT SIXTEEN 1-OUNCE FREEZER CUBES**

1 parsnip, peeled and cut into ½-inch dice

1 medium sweet potato, peeled and cut into ½-inch dice

1 golden beet, peeled and cut into ½-inch dice

1 teaspoon melted coconut oil or avocado oil

½ teaspoon dried thyme

½ to 1 cup filtered water, plus more to thin to desired consistency

1   Preheat the oven to 400°F. Line a baking sheet with parchment paper.

2   Put the parsnip, sweet potato, and golden beet on the prepared baking sheet. Drizzle with the oil, and sprinkle with the thyme. With clean hands, mix together until evenly coated.

3   Transfer the baking sheet to the oven, and bake for 30 minutes, stirring halfway through, or until fork-tender. Remove from the oven. Transfer to a blender.

4   Add the water and purée until smooth, adding more water to thin to your desired consistency.

Storage: Divide into ice cube trays, freeze overnight, and transfer to an airtight zip-top bag or glass container. Freeze for up to 6 months. You can alternatively save some in a glass jar in the refrigerator for up to 3 days and divide the rest to freeze.

Tip: You could use a carrot instead of a parsnip. And for a non-vegetarian version, you can try using bone broth instead of water.

7 TO 8 MONTHS

Banana Coconut Custard

PREP TIME: 5 minutes **COOK TIME:** 45 minutes

FREEZER-FRIENDLY • DAIRY-FREE OPTION • GLUTEN-FREE • NUT-FREE • VEGAN OPTION • VEGETARIAN

This little treat is likely to be a favorite, and it will provide the saturated fats and good cholesterol necessary for your baby's brain health. The egg yolks offer essential choline for healthy cell membranes, loads of vitamins and minerals, and amino acids. Coconut milk is high in lauric acid, which the body uses to make monolaurin, a strong antiviral component. **MAKES 12 MINI CUSTARDS**

¼ cup (½ stick) grass-fed, unsalted butter or ghee, plus more for greasing

1 (15-ounce) can full-fat coconut cream

6 large egg yolks

1 teaspoon alcohol-free vanilla extract

1 ripe banana, with spots

1 Preheat the oven to 325°F. Grease a mini muffin pan.

2 In a small skillet, melt the butter over low heat. Remove from the heat. Transfer to a blender.

3 Add the coconut cream, egg yolks, vanilla, and banana. Blend for about 30 seconds, or until smooth.

4 Pour the banana batter into the cups of the prepared pan.

5 Fill a 9 x 13-inch baking dish three-quarters full with water, and set the muffin pan inside.

6 Carefully transfer the baking dish to the oven, and bake for about 45 minutes, or until firm and set. Remove from the oven.

7 Let the custard cool in the pan. Scoop out and serve.

Storage: Store in the refrigerator, covered, for up to 3 days.

Tip: To make this dairy-free, use coconut oil instead of ghee.

Leek, Potato, and Pea Purée

PREP TIME: 10 minutes **COOK TIME:** 10 minutes

FREEZER-FRIENDLY · **DAIRY-FREE** · **GLUTEN-FREE** · **NUT-FREE** · **VEGAN** · **VEGETARIAN**

Full disclosure: This flavor combo is so tasty that I ended up eating half of it while making it for my youngest. White and yellow potatoes are considered by some food experts to be a nightshade, so it's best to skip this recipe for a sensitive baby and wait until after 12 months of age to introduce them. When they're ready, this one is sure to be a hit! **MAKES ABOUT SIXTEEN 1-OUNCE FREEZER CUBES**

7 TO 8 MONTHS

1 ¼ cups filtered water

⅓ cup frozen peas

½ cup diced (1 inch) yellow potato

⅓ cup finely chopped, well-washed leek

⅛ teaspoon ground cumin

⅛ teaspoon dried oregano

⅛ teaspoon garlic powder

1   In a medium saucepan, combine the water, peas, potato, leek, cumin, oregano, and garlic powder.

2   Bring to a boil, then reduce the heat to a simmer. Cover with a lid, and cook for 5 to 7 minutes, or until the vegetables have cooked through.

3   Remove from the heat. Let cool with the lid off. Transfer to a blender, and purée to your desired consistency.

Storage: Divide into ice cube trays, freeze overnight, and transfer to an airtight zip-top bag or glass container. Freeze for up to 6 months. You can alternatively save some in the refrigerator in a glass jar and divide the rest to freeze.

Tip: This recipe is easy to double if you want to freeze more. I encourage you to try it unpuréed the next time you make it, and offer it as finger food. And for a non-vegetarian version, try using bone broth instead of water.

You can also use any leftover purée to make potato pancakes. Just grease a skillet and use it as you would pancake batter, for a savory pancake alternative.

Beef and Sweet Potato Purée

PREP TIME: 10 minutes **COOK TIME:** 25 to 30 minutes
FREEZER-FRIENDLY · **DAIRY-FREE** · **GLUTEN-FREE** · **NUT-FREE**

Is it time for some meat and potatoes? Start here! Sweet potato offers that good-for-you beta-carotene, and when combined with steak, it makes for a savory, filling meal your baby will love. Adding beef to your baby's diet in any form is a sure way to increase their heme iron, which is the most absorbable type. **MAKES ABOUT 2 CUPS**

1 cup filtered water, plus more to thin to desired consistency

¼ pound grass-fed beef top sirloin, diced

1 sweet potato, cut into 1-inch dice

1 teaspoon fresh thyme leaves

2 tablespoons coconut oil

1 In a medium saucepan, bring the water to a boil.

2 Add the beef, sweet potato, and thyme. Reduce the heat to low, and simmer for 20 to 25 minutes, or until the beef is cooked and sweet potato is tender. Remove from the heat. Transfer to a blender.

3 Add the coconut oil and purée until smooth, adding more water to thin to your desired consistency.

Storage: Keep a portion in an airtight glass container in the refrigerator for up to 3 days or freeze leftovers for up to 3 months.

Tip: You can try using bone broth instead of water, and if you're comfortable with dairy, you can use ghee or grass-fed butter instead of coconut oil.

Kiwi, Pear, and Spinach Purée

PREP TIME: 5 to 10 minutes **COOK TIME:** 10 to 15 minutes
FREEZER-FRIENDLY · DAIRY-FREE · GLUTEN-FREE · NUT-FREE · VEGAN · VEGETARIAN

This green combo offers a little sweet and a taste of spinach for your baby. It's best to offer these three foods separately first to make sure your baby tolerates them all. Kiwi, banana, avocado, and latex are all in the same allergen category, so if your baby is sensitive to any of these things, skip this recipe. Also, spinach is a great choice for your organic dollar, as it's on the Dirty Dozen list (page 12). **MAKES ABOUT 1 CUP**

1 ripe pear, peeled and cut into 1-inch dice

1 cup fresh spinach

1 kiwi, peeled

1 Steam the pear as described in Spiced Pear and Prune Purée (page 118), leaving the water boiling and the steaming basket in the saucepan. Transfer the pear to a blender.

2 Put the spinach in the basket. Tightly cover and steam for about 2 minutes, or until wilted. Remove from the heat.

3 Add the steamed spinach and kiwi to the blender with the pear. Purée until smooth, adding a splash of filtered water as needed.

Storage: Divide into ice cube trays, freeze overnight, and transfer to an airtight zip bag or glass container for up to 6 months. You can alternatively save some in a glass jar in the refrigerator for up to 3 days and divide the rest to freeze.

Tip: You can double this if you want to make a bigger freezer stash.

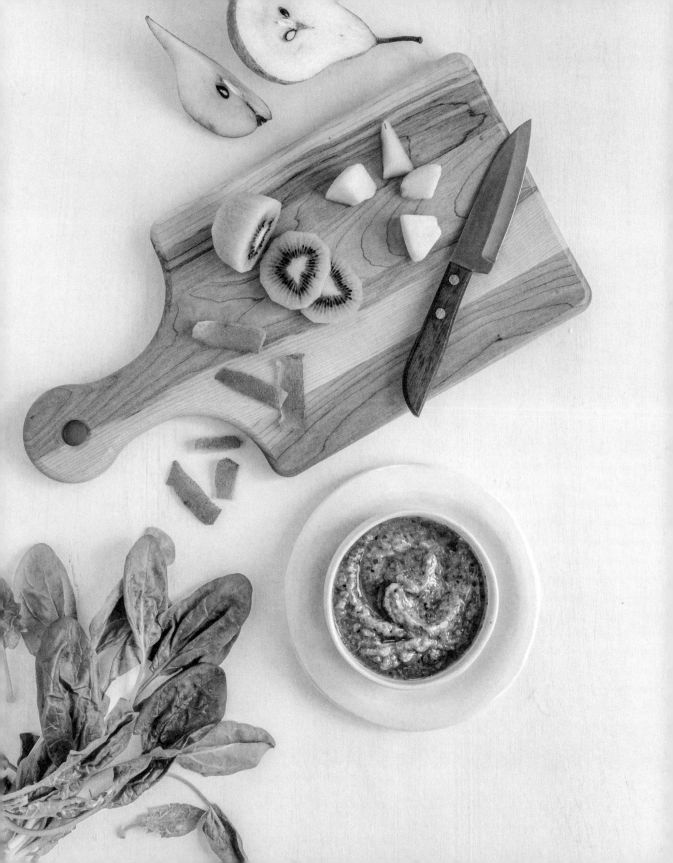

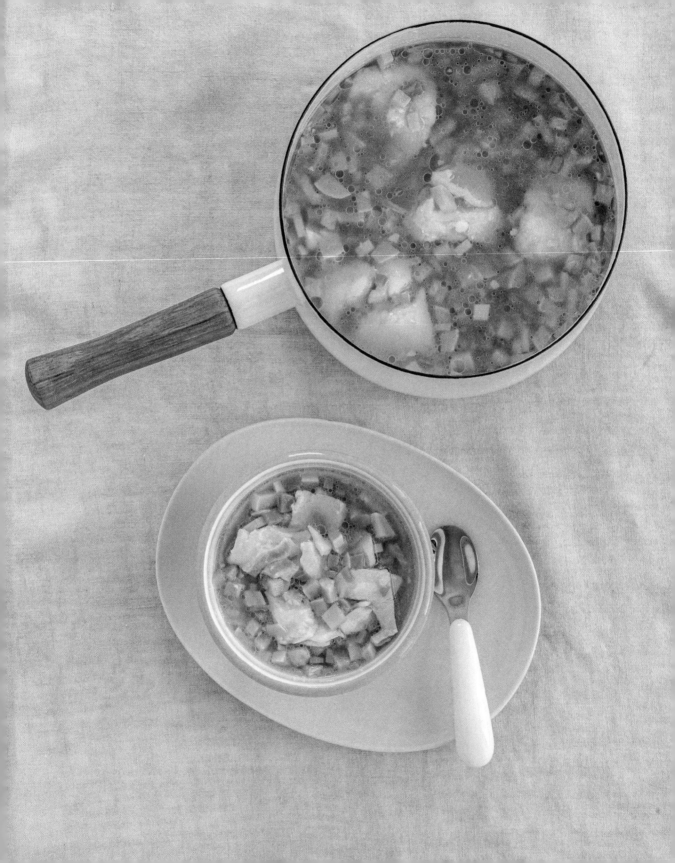

Seven

Chunky Meals & Finger Foods

8 TO 12 MONTHS

Chunky Meals

Minty Watermelon
Breakfast Bowl *130*

Sweet Potato Yogurt
Breakfast Bowl *131*

Blueberry, Banana, and
Avocado Bowl *132*

Homemade Yogurt
with Berries *134*

Easy Banana Pancakes *137*

Lemony Chicken and
Carrot Soup *138*

Pumpkin and Cod Soup *139*

Poached Cod with Carrots
and Squash *140*

Avocado and Mackerel
Salad *141*

Coconut Chicken Curry with
Carrots and Potatoes *142*

Egg Drop Soup with
Chicken *143*

Steak and Veggie
Stir-Fry *144*

Turkey and Zucchini
Herb Bowl *145*

Roasted Rainbow Spuds *146*

Sweet Potato Pancakes *147*

Finger Foods

Wiggly Jigglers *148*

Banana Mini Muffins *149*

Hooray for Hummus Dip *150*

Roasted Cauliflower
with Peanut Dip *151*

Sweet Potato Crackers *152*

Sweet Potato Balls *153*

Pork Sausage Patties *153*

Italian Cloud Bread *154*

Chicken and Black
Bean Quesadilla *156*

Mushroom and Black
Olive Pizza *158*

Veggie Marinara *160*

Healthy Smash Cake *161*

Around 8 to 10 months, many babies start to develop the pincer grasp. This is exemplified by touching one finger to a thumb to hold something. It is helping to develop the action of grasping. Babies do this as a means of exploration, and it is so much fun to watch! They also start to put *everything* in their mouth around this age, so if your baby has not been too interested in self-feeding yet, they may be from now on! This is a perfect time to begin finger foods. Some of the soft fruits and veggies in this next meal plan can be puréed. This is an especially important time to supervise, as you'll be watching for how baby navigates different sizes and textures, and of course making sure your baby isn't filling their mouth with too much. If they do, it's important not to intervene by trying to put your fingers in their mouth; rather, teach them by calmly saying "that's too much food" and show them how to open their mouth and push their tongue out, saying "ah" repeatedly.

WHAT TO EXPECT

Around 8 to 9 months, you will start to establish a more consistent pattern of feeding, rather than offering random tastes of things. You'll still want to avoid any strict schedule. Foods should vary in texture and include some very soft, mushy lumps. For most babies, it's appropriate to offer small chunks of finger foods along with some purées. Continue offering easy-grip spoons and forks, but don't expect them to be used. It's more about practicing and feeling free to use their hands for the full sensory experience. A few recipes in this chapter will include gluten-free flours like coconut flour, almond flour, and oat flour, as baby does not yet have large amounts of amylase (a digestive enzyme) to break down grain starches at this age.

How Much to Feed
2 tablespoons to ½ cup, following baby's lead

When to Feed
About 2 to 3 meals per day. Every baby's eating rhythm will look different, but an example at 8 to 9 months could be: wake up, nurse/bottle, mid-morning meal, nurse/bottle before an afternoon nap, dinner with the family, and nurse/bottle before bed. Babies tend to begin eating 3 small meals a day at different times, but usually at around 9 to 12 months.

What to Drink
Breast milk, formula, bone broth, and water are the only appropriate liquids to offer your baby at this age. At 12 months, you can introduce cow's milk if you desire, but it is not required.

First-Time Parent Tip

When your baby turns 12 months, many nursing moms believe they must introduce cow's milk. However, if you're nursing, your toddler is already getting the most nutritious milk available and there is no requirement to introduce cow's milk (see Introducing Milk at 12 Months, page 163).

Minty Watermelon Breakfast Bowl

PREP TIME: 15 minutes

FREEZER-FRIENDLY · **DAIRY-FREE** · **GLUTEN-FREE** · **NUT-FREE OPTION** · **VEGAN OPTION** · **VEGETARIAN**

Watermelon is a juicy hit for most kids. Served over coconut chia mousse, it makes for a perfect protein-and-fat breakfast bowl, introducing your little one to the flavor of mint. Adults will love this juicy, refreshing, and summery combination, too! Try offering watermelon in different cuts, such as ruler-thick slices, for your baby to practice grabbing and picking up. **MAKES ABOUT 2 CUPS**

1 cup finely diced seedless watermelon

1 teaspoon minced fresh mint

½ teaspoon fresh lemon juice

¼ teaspoon olive oil

1 cup Chia Seed Mousse (page 176)

In a small bowl, combine the watermelon, mint, lemon juice, and olive oil. Stir, and serve over chia seed mousse.

Storage: Keep in an airtight glass container in the refrigerator for up to 3 days.

Tip: You could serve this over Homemade Yogurt (page 134) or store-bought, full-fat, plain yogurt instead of coconut chia seed mousse.

8 TO 12 MONTHS

Sweet Potato Yogurt Breakfast Bowl

PREP TIME: 5 to 10 minutes
GLUTEN-FREE · **VEGETARIAN**

This breakfast bowl is a perfect blend of sweet and savory, giving your little one the energy they need for the morning ahead. Sometimes babies and toddlers like their food deconstructed so they can experience flavors and textures individually. Other times, they like to explore the combination of foods together. Serve this bowl to a baby who has already been introduced to all these ingredients, closer to 11 months of age. **MAKES ABOUT 1 CUP**

½ cup full-fat, plain yogurt

½ teaspoon alcohol-free vanilla extract

⅛ teaspoon ground cinnamon

¼ teaspoon chia seeds

¼ teaspoon flax meal

1 dollop of almond butter, plus more for garnish

½ to 1 teaspoon maple syrup

¼ cup fresh blueberries, smashed

¼ cup diced sweet potato, roasted or steamed

Storage: Keep in an airtight glass container in the refrigerator for up to 3 days.

Tip: You can garnish with nut butter or seed butter, such as sunflower, to avoid allergen exposure. For babies more than 12 months old who have been introduced to honey, you could substitute honey for maple syrup.

1 In a medium bowl, combine the yogurt, vanilla, cinnamon, chia seeds, flax meal, almond butter, and maple syrup. Mix well.

2 Add the blueberries and sweet potato.

Blueberry, Banana, and Avocado Bowl

PREP TIME: 10 minutes

BLW · **DAIRY-FREE** · **GLUTEN-FREE** · **NUT-FREE** · **VEGAN** · **VEGETARIAN**

This recipe is great for a baby around 10 or 11 months old who has been introduced to all of these foods separately. It's a perfect way to practice picking up different foods, combining them together in one meal so baby can experience the flavor combination and different textures. The optional flax meal provides omega-3 fatty acids, fiber, and more, keeping baby full and healthy. **MAKES 1 TO 2 CUPS**

¼ ripe avocado, pitted and peeled

½ banana, peeled

1 to 2 teaspoons flax meal (optional)

¼ cup smashed blueberries

1   Cut the avocado into slices the length and width of your finger.

2   Cut the banana like the avocado, making 4 long slices that are easy to grasp with the whole hand.

3   Dust the avocado and banana with the flax meal (if using) to coat evenly. This helps give your baby a better grip. Transfer to a bowl.

4   Add the blueberries and serve.

Storage: This bowl doesn't keep that well in the refrigerator, but if you have leftovers, consider making them into a smoothie.

Tip: Want to make this into a smoothie for your baby? Just add all the ingredients to a blender with about ¼ cup filtered water or plain yogurt (if dairy has been introduced) and a few ice cubes, and blend on high. Serve with a straw so your baby can practice sipping.

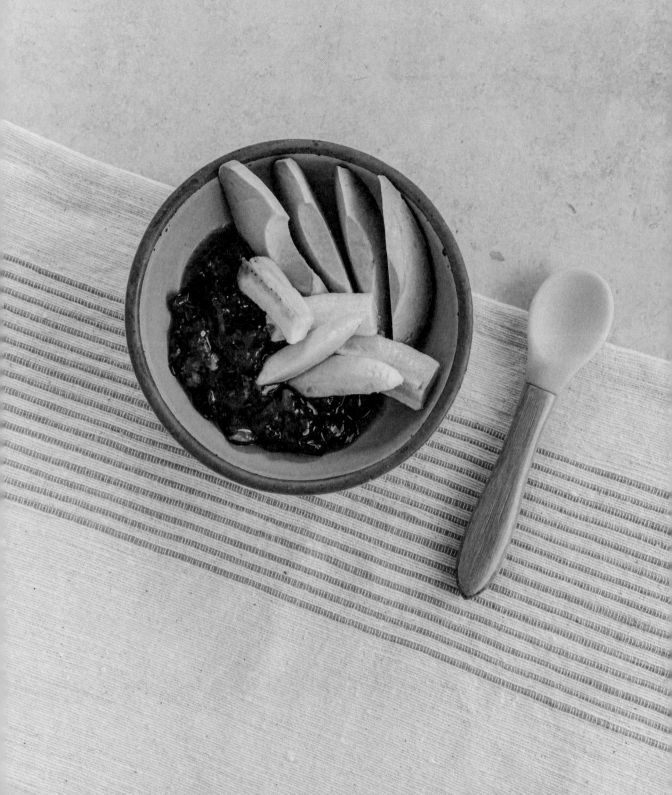

Homemade Yogurt with Berries

PREP TIME: 5 minutes, plus 16 to 28 hours for the yogurt to incubate and set
COOK TIME: 10 to 15 minutes
GLUTEN-FREE · **NUT-FREE** · **VEGETARIAN**

Around 9 months of age, the introduction of yogurt is appropriate for babies who do not have signs of dairy sensitivity. Cultured dairy such as yogurt is probiotic-rich, giving the gut lots of good bacteria. The most valuable and nutrient-rich type of milk is raw milk from a clean source. Many states allow the sale of raw milk in retail stores, but other states have restrictions. If you have access to raw milk, it's preferred. If not, a local milk made by a "vat pasteurization" process is best, not "ultra pasteurized." Make sure to get whole milk for the most nutrition. Homemade yogurt also yields a protein called whey, which can be used to for soaking grains (see page 36). You will need one 1-quart sterilized canning jar for this. **MAKES ABOUT 4 CUPS**

8 TO 12 MONTHS

1 quart whole milk

2 tablespoons plain, whole-milk yogurt

A few tablespoons maple syrup (optional)

¼ cup berries, already introduced in the diet

1 In a large stainless-steel pan, heat the milk over medium heat until it reaches 180°F. Remove from the heat. Transfer to the canning jar. Let cool to 115°F, by either setting on the counter or placing in a cool water bath.

2 Add the yogurt and lightly stir.

3 Transfer the jar to the oven, and let incubate with the oven light on for 12 to 24 hours. The longer the yogurt incubates, the tangier it will be. The heat from your oven light will provide a consistent heat. You could, alternatively, put it in another warm place in your home.

4   Refrigerate the yogurt until it is set
and cold.

5   Pour off and reserve the whey (the liquid
on top), or strain with a cheesecloth (or
clean, thin cotton kitchen towel) for a
thicker yogurt. Reserve the whey in the
refrigerator in a clean glass jar for up to
2 months, and use it for future soaking
recipes, if desired.

6   Add the maple syrup (if using).

7   When ready to serve the yogurt, smash
the berries. This helps prevent choking.

Storage: Keep in an airtight glass
container in the refrigerator for up to
2 weeks.

Tip: Alternatively, you could use
goat's milk.

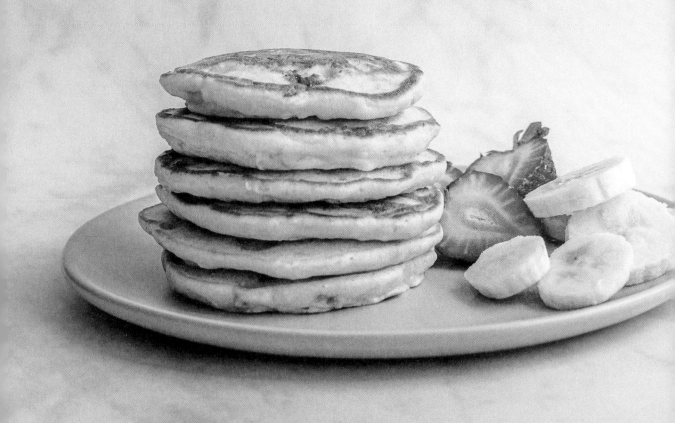

Easy Banana Pancakes

PREP TIME: 5 minutes **COOK TIME:** 5 to 10 minutes
FREEZER-FRIENDLY · **DAIRY-FREE** · **GLUTEN-FREE** · **NUT-FREE** · **VEGETARIAN**

You're not likely to get much pushback on this dish. In fact, it'll probably be a recipe your little one enjoys for years to come! This recipe uses egg yolk, but if your baby is 12 months or older, you could use a whole egg instead. I usually double (or triple) pancake recipes to freeze in bulk. **SERVES 4**

1 ripe banana, peeled

2 egg yolks or 1 large egg (see head note)

½ cup coconut flour

1 teaspoon aluminum-free baking powder

⅛ teaspoon ground cinnamon (optional)

Coconut oil, for greasing

1 In a medium bowl, mash the banana.

2 Add the egg yolks, flour, baking powder, and cinnamon (if using). Whisk just until the ingredients come together; do not overmix.

3 Grease a medium nonstick skillet, and preheat over medium-low heat.

4 Scoop about ¼ cup of batter into the skillet. Cook for 3 to 4 minutes on each side, or until golden. Remove from the heat.

Storage: Keep in an airtight glass container in the refrigerator for up to 3 days or up to 3 months in the freezer.

Tip: You can get creative and replace 1 tablespoon of the banana with pumpkin or another purée. Around 12 to 18 months, you can use whole-wheat or all-purpose flour instead of coconut flour (see What to Expect, page 129).

Lemony Chicken and Carrot Soup

PREP TIME: 10 to 15 minutes **COOK TIME:** 25 to 30 minutes
FREEZER-FRIENDLY · **DAIRY-FREE OPTION** · **GLUTEN-FREE** · **NUT-FREE**

Although this is a soup, it's a great dish to serve as finger food. The soup contains a yummy blend of soft-cooked veggies and chicken for your adventurous eater. It's perfect for a baby who has already been introduced to all of these foods and is practicing the pincer grasp. Make sure all foods are cut into small, soft, mashable finger foods, and add just a little broth. **SERVES 8 GENEROUSLY**

3 tablespoons grass-fed, unsalted butter

2 boneless, skinless chicken breasts

¼ teaspoon freshly ground black pepper

1 yellow onion, diced

2 carrots, diced

1 small green zucchini, diced

1 teaspoon dried thyme

1 ¼ quarts bone broth

Juice of 1 lemon

1   In a large pot, melt 1 tablespoon of butter over medium heat.

2   Add the chicken and cook for 3 to 4 minutes on each side, or until cooked through. Transfer to a plate.

3   Melt the remaining 2 tablespoons of butter in the pot.

4   Add the onion, carrots, zucchini, and thyme. Cook for 3 to 4 minutes, or until they begin to soften.

5   Add the bone broth, scraping any browned bits from the bottom of the pot. Bring to a boil.

6   Meanwhile, chop the chicken into finger food–size chunks. Once the soup comes to a rolling boil, stir in the chicken.

7   Reduce the heat to a simmer, and cook for 10 to 12 minutes, or until the vegetables are very tender. Remove from the heat.

8   Stir in the lemon juice.

Storage: Keep in an airtight glass container in the refrigerator for up to 3 days or up to 3 months in the freezer.

Tip: You can substitute coconut oil for butter for a dairy-free option.

Pumpkin and Cod Soup

PREP TIME: 15 to 20 minutes **COOK TIME:** 50 to 55 minutes

FREEZER-FRIENDLY · **DAIRY-FREE OPTION** · **GLUTEN-FREE** · **NUT-FREE**

Pumpkin enjoys a wide nutritional profile, enhancing bones and teeth, immunity, eyesight, and more. Adding fish provides a meal rich with omega-3s and vitamins to nourish your little one. If you're making this recipe when your little one is less than 12 months old, use coconut cream instead. **SERVES 4 TO 6**

4 tablespoons ghee or coconut oil

½ medium onion, diced

½ medium pumpkin, peeled, seeded, and finely diced

2 (4-ounce) cod fillets

3 cups bone broth

Freshly ground black pepper to taste

¼ cup heavy cream (or canned coconut cream if less than 12 months old)

1 In a medium saucepan, melt 3 tablespoons of ghee over medium-high heat.

2 Add the onion and sauté, stirring occasionally for 5 to 6 minutes, or until translucent.

3 Add the pumpkin and cook, stirring occasionally for about 15 minutes, or until browned.

4 Meanwhile, in a small saucepan, melt the remaining 1 tablespoon of ghee over medium-high heat.

5 Add the cod to the small saucepan. Sauté for 2 to 3 minutes on each side, or until easily flaked with a fork and cooked through. Remove from the heat. Transfer to a plate.

6 To the medium saucepan, add the bone broth, bring to a simmer, and cook for about 30 minutes, or until the pumpkin is mushy. Remove from the heat and let cool a bit. Transfer to a blender, and purée until smooth. Season with pepper to taste. Return to the pan.

7 Add the cream. Bring to a boil over low heat. Remove from the heat.

8 Flake one quarter to one half of a cod fillet into the soup per serving.

Storage: Keep the cod and soup in separate glass containers in the refrigerator for up to 3 days.

Tip: You can use sweet potato instead of pumpkin here.

Poached Cod with Carrots and Squash

PREP TIME: 15 to 20 minutes **COOK TIME:** 30 to 35 minutes

FREEZER-FRIENDLY · DAIRY-FREE OPTION · GLUTEN-FREE · NUT-FREE

The texture of these foods makes for a soft, easy-to-eat meal for your baby. This savory flavor combination is one of my favorites. If your child hasn't been interested in fish yet, try serving something they like, such as carrots or squash, alongside the fish. This may increase the chance they'll try it on the first go-round! SERVES 4 TO 6

8 TO 12 MONTHS

3 tablespoons coconut oil, ghee, or grass-fed, unsalted butter

1 tablespoon minced white onion

1 tablespoon minced garlic

Sprinkle of turmeric

1 tablespoon grated ginger (optional)

2 carrots, finely diced

1 yellow squash, finely diced

3 to 4 cups bone broth

4 (4-ounce) cod fillets

1   In a large skillet, melt the coconut oil over medium heat.

2   Add the onion, garlic, turmeric, and ginger (if using). Sauté for 3 to 5 minutes, or until the garlic and onion are soft and translucent.

3   Add the carrots and squash. Cook for 5 to 7 minutes, or until soft.

4   Add the bone broth and simmer for 10 minutes.

5   Add the cod, immersing it completely in the broth. Cover with a lid, and cook for 6 to 8 minutes, or until easily flaked with a fork and cooked through. Remove from the heat.

Storage: Keep in an airtight glass container in the refrigerator for up to 3 days.

Tip: Haddock is a good substitute for cod.

Avocado and Mackerel Salad

PREP TIME: 5 to 10 minutes
DAIRY-FREE · GLUTEN-FREE · NUT-FREE

If you haven't tried mackerel, it has a similar taste to tuna. Babies under 12 months old need about 500mg DPA and EPA daily—two fatty acids that are found in fish like mackerel. Fats like these help your baby's brain develop properly. Mackerel is considered a "SMASH" fish (sardines, mackerel, anchovies, salmon, and herring), otherwise known as the best fish for you due to the low mercury and high omega-3 levels (see page 16). This may sound totally new, but this is basically tuna salad with mackerel. Give it a try! SERVES 3 TO 4

1 (4-ounce) can mackerel, drained

2 to 3 tablespoons avocado oil– or olive oil– based mayonnaise

Pinch of freshly ground black pepper

½ ripe avocado, halved, pitted, peeled, and sliced

In a small bowl, combine the mackerel, mayonnaise, pepper, and avocado. Smash to form a chunky, moist mixture.

Storage: Keep in a glass jar in the refrigerator for up to 3 days.

Tip: You can add shredded carrot or minced celery for babies older than 15 months, and you can substitute canned salmon for mackerel. Also, a few shakes of curry powder make for a good variation in flavor.

Coconut Chicken Curry with Carrots and Potatoes

PREP TIME: 15 to 20 minutes **COOK TIME:** 20 to 25 minutes

FREEZER-FRIENDLY · DAIRY-FREE OPTION · GLUTEN-FREE · NUT-FREE

This nutrient-packed meal is likely to become a family favorite. You can serve it over soaked rice (see page 36), or make cauliflower rice to serve alongside this dish. Yellow curry powder aids in digestion and has antibacterial properties. Make sure the ingredients are cooked super soft and served in small chunks, easy for your baby to pick up and mash between fingers and gums. **SERVES 6 TO 8**

1 to 2 pounds boneless, skinless chicken, cut into ½-inch dice

4 ½ to 5 teaspoons mild yellow curry powder

½ to 1 teaspoon freshly ground black pepper

2 tablespoons grass-fed, unsalted butter or coconut oil

1 onion, diced

2 carrots, chopped

1 large sweet potato, cut into ½-inch dice

2 (15-ounce) cans full-fat coconut milk

1 teaspoon ground ginger

2 teaspoons chopped garlic

2 cups fresh spinach

1 In a large bowl, toss together the chicken, curry powder, and pepper. Set aside.

2 In a saucepan, melt the butter over medium heat.

3 Add the onion and sauté for 5 minutes.

4 Add the carrots and sweet potato. Cook for 2 to 3 minutes.

5 Add the coconut milk, ginger, garlic, and chicken. Cover with a lid, and cook for about 15 minutes.

6 Fold in the spinach. Remove from the heat. Serve over rice if 15 months or older (see page 36 for how to prepare for a baby).

Storage: Keep in an airtight glass container in the refrigerator for up to 3 to 4 days or in the freezer for up to 3 months.

Tip: You can double this recipe and freeze half to pull out on a night when you need something quick and nourishing.

8 TO 12 MONTHS

Egg Drop Soup with Chicken

PREP TIME: 15 minutes **COOK TIME:** 30 to 35 minutes

DAIRY-FREE · GLUTEN-FREE · NUT-FREE

This soup just like chicken noodle soup, warms the soul, and I love how little prep it takes. Whip this up during the fall season to keep your family well and warm. Its immune-boosting properties are abundant in every ingredient! **SERVES 8**

Filtered water

2 boneless, skinless chicken breasts (about 1 ¼ pounds)

1 onion, chopped

4 cups chopped carrots, cut in ¼-inch disks (about 8 carrots)

4 celery stalks, chopped

2 teaspoons garlic powder

¼ teaspoon freshly ground black pepper, or to taste

5 large eggs

1 Fill a medium pot with 4 cups water. Add the chicken. Bring to a gentle boil over medium heat. Remove from the heat. Flip the chicken over, cover with a lid, and leave it in the pot for 10 minutes, or until cooked through. Transfer the chicken to a cutting board. Once cool enough to handle, chop it into bite-size pieces.

2 To the water in the pot, add the onion, carrots, and celery. Bring to a boil. Cook for 10 to 12 minutes, or until the vegetables are soft.

3 Add the chopped chicken, garlic powder, and pepper.

4 Reduce the heat to a simmer. Break the eggs one by one into the pot, stirring vigorously after each addition. Simmer for 1 minute or so, and remove from the heat. Season with pepper to taste.

Storage: Keep in an airtight glass container in the refrigerator for up to 3 days.

Steak and Veggie Stir-Fry

PREP TIME: 15 to 20 minutes **COOK TIME:** 10 to 15 minutes

FREEZER-FRIENDLY · **DAIRY-FREE** · **GLUTEN-FREE OPTION** · **NUT-FREE**

It's fun to involve the kids with this meal because as you chop the vegetables, they can transfer them into a big bowl until it's time to cook. Even a young kiddo around 18 months old can help with prep work. When kids help in the kitchen, it increases their interest in food preparation, the meal itself, and in food in general. **SERVES 4 TO 6**

8 TO 12 MONTHS

2 tablespoons olive oil

1 onion, chopped

2 bell peppers, cored and chopped

1 large zucchini or yellow squash, cut into half-moons

1 cup broccoli florets

1 cup cauliflower florets

1 cup shredded carrot

¼ low-sodium soy sauce

1 pound flank steak, cut into ½-inch strips

1 tablespoon coarsely chopped garlic

2 tablespoons sesame oil

1 In a large skillet, heat the olive oil over medium-high heat.

2 Add the onion, peppers, zucchini, broccoli, cauliflower, carrot, and soy sauce. Cover with a lid and cook for 8 to 10 minutes, or until the vegetables are soft. Transfer to a large serving bowl.

3 Add the beef and garlic. Cook until the beef is cooked to your desired doneness. Remove from the heat. Stir into the vegetable mixture.

4 Add the sesame oil, and toss. Serve over rice, if 15 months or older (see page 36 for how to prepare for baby).

Storage: Keep everything together in an airtight glass container in the refrigerator for up to 3 days.

Tip: You can use any vegetables in your refrigerator that need to be used up. Try cabbage, Brussels sprouts, more peppers, or snap peas. You just need about 4 cups of vegetables. For a gluten-free option, you can use tamari or coconut aminos instead of soy sauce.

Turkey and Zucchini Herb Bowl

PREP TIME: 10 to 20 minutes **COOK TIME:** 15 to 20 minutes
FREEZER-FRIENDLY · DAIRY-FREE · GLUTEN-FREE · NUT-FREE

This recipe is super quick to whip up and a favorite meal for a weekly rotation. It's great for little fingers to pick up, beginning around 9 months of age, and packed with nutrition. Adding herbs to the dish adds variety and new flavors for your child to experience. SERVES ABOUT 4

1 large zucchini or 3 small zucchini, peeled

1 pound ground turkey

¼ cup fresh basil, minced, or 1 teaspoon dried

2 tablespoons fresh oregano or 1 teaspoon dried

1 tablespoon fresh parsley, minced, or 2 teaspoons dried

1 tablespoon olive oil or avocado oil

4 teaspoons minced garlic

1 yellow onion, diced

⅓ cup marinara sauce

1   Cut the zucchini into half-moons, then cut in half again.

2   Put the turkey in a medium nonstick saucepan, and cook over medium heat, breaking up the meat, for 4 to 6 minutes, or until cooked through.

3   If using dried basil, oregano, and parsley, add them now.

4   Add the oil, garlic, and onion. Cook for 3 to 4 minutes, or just until the onion begins to soften.

5   Add the zucchini and marinara sauce. Cover with a lid and cook for 5 to 7 minutes, or until the zucchini is tender. Remove from the heat.

6   If using fresh basil, oregano, and parsley, stir them in now.

Storage: Keep in an airtight glass container in the refrigerator for up to 3 days.

Tip: You could use yellow summer squash instead of zucchini. This mixture is super tasty stuffed inside a sweet potato or butternut squash.

Roasted Rainbow Spuds

PREP TIME: 10 to 15 minutes **COOK TIME:** 40 minutes
DAIRY-FREE · **GLUTEN-FREE** · **NUT-FREE** · **VEGAN** · **VEGETARIAN**

Different colors deliver different nutritional benefits, even when those colors all come from one food! Here, we'll capitalize on the variety of potatoes available. Both the beautiful colors and the shape of these beauties make eating fun. Serve as a finger food for your baby, alongside a dip of plain Greek yogurt. **SERVES 4 TO 8**

8 TO 12 MONTHS

**2 purple potatoes or purple sweet potatoes,
cut into ½-inch half-moons**

2 sweet potatoes, cut into ½-inch half-moons

3 tablespoons avocado oil or melted coconut oil

1 teaspoon freshly ground black pepper

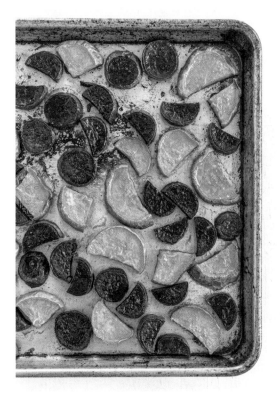

1   Preheat the oven to 400°F.

2   In a large bowl, combine the potatoes, sweet potatoes, oil, and pepper. Toss, then arrange flat on a baking sheet.

3   Transfer the baking sheet to the oven, and bake for 20 minutes.

4   Raise the heat to 425°F. Bake for 20 minutes or until soft. Remove from the oven.

   Storage: Keep in an airtight glass container in the refrigerator for up to 3 days.

Sweet Potato Pancakes

PREP TIME: 5 minutes **COOK TIME:** 5 to 10 minutes
FREEZER-FRIENDLY · **DAIRY-FREE** · **GLUTEN-FREE** · **NUT-FREE** · **VEGETARIAN**

Here's a twist on the traditional pancake. More like a hash brown, it's made with sweet potato and warm spices. This recipe is best for a baby around 12 months of age because it contains whole eggs. I would recommend first introducing your baby to a whole egg by itself, unless they have already been introduced to every ingredient in this recipe. MAKES ABOUT EIGHT 2-INCH PANCAKES

½ cup mashed, cooked, peeled sweet potato

2 large eggs

¾ teaspoon ground cinnamon

¼ teaspoon ground ginger

¼ teaspoon ground nutmeg

Coconut oil, for frying

Grass-fed butter, for serving

1 In a medium bowl, mix together the sweet potato and eggs until very smooth.

2 Add the cinnamon, ginger, and nutmeg. Mix to combine.

3 In a medium saucepan, heat a thin layer of coconut oil over medium heat.

4 Spoon 1 to 2 tablespoons of batter in the pan, and repeat to make eight 2-inch pancakes. Small pancakes flip more easily.

5 Reduce the heat to medium-low. Cook the pancakes for 2 to 3 minutes on each side. Top with butter.

Storage: Keep in an airtight glass container in the refrigerator for up to 3 days or up to 3 months in the freezer.

Wiggly Jigglers

PREP TIME: 10 minutes, plus 3 hours to set
DAIRY-FREE · GLUTEN-FREE · NUT-FREE

Boxed flavored gelatin mixes are loaded with artificial dye and sugar, but this homemade version offers an easy, nutritious alternative. Unprocessed gelatin like we use here contains important amino acids and is nourishing to the gut. I flavor it with real grape or apple juice because it puts a healthy spin on a fun food. Grape juice supposedly can change the pH of your stomach to prevent a stomach bug. There is no official study I can find, but I am speaking from experience along with testimonies from lots of moms in the medical field. Plus, it's a good excuse for a fun-colored jiggler. **SERVES 16 GENEROUSLY**

Coconut oil, for greasing

3 ½ cups no-added-sugar apple juice or grape juice (not from concentrate)

2 tablespoons unflavored gelatin powder

½ cup boiling filtered water

1 Grease an 8 x 8-inch pan with coconut oil.

2 In a medium bowl, combine ½ cup of juice and the gelatin powder. Whisk it quickly and vigorously before it sets.

3 Immediately add the boiling water and whisk until combined.

4 Add the remaining 3 cups of juice.

5 Pour the mixture into the prepared pan. Refrigerate for at least 3 hours to set. Cut into cubes and serve as finger food.

Storage: Keep in an airtight glass container in the refrigerator for up to 3 days.

Tip: It helps to have the liquids (juice, boiling water) already measured out in separate cups and ready to add. You can also cut this recipe in half for a smaller batch.

Banana Mini Muffins

PREP TIME: 5 to 10 minutes **COOK TIME:** 20 to 25 minutes
DAIRY-FREE · GLUTEN-FREE · NUT-FREE · VEGAN OPTION · VEGETARIAN

These are ideal to whip up ahead and reach for during the week. Depending on your baby's chewing development and eating skills, some babies may need to have foods like these served a special way, since bread textures can clump together in the mouth and become a choking hazard. Generally, from 8 to 10 months, these muffins would be best served broken into pieces. For 11 to 12 months, offering a muffin in 2 halves may be more appropriate. MAKES 12 TO 15 MINI MUFFINS

½ cup (1 stick) grass-fed, unsalted butter or coconut oil, melted, plus more for greasing

½ cup maple syrup or honey (only use honey if over 12 months old)

1 cup mashed ripe bananas

2 teaspoons alcohol-free vanilla extract

2 cups oat flour (see Tip)

1 teaspoon baking soda

1 teaspoon aluminum-free baking powder

2 tablespoons flax meal (optional)

½ cup chopped walnuts (optional)

1 Preheat the oven to 350°F. Grease a mini muffin pan.

2 In a large bowl, whisk the butter and maple syrup until thoroughly mixed.

3 Add the bananas, vanilla, oat flour, baking soda, baking powder, and flax meal (if using). Mix just until combined.

4 Fold in the walnuts (if using). Pour into the prepared muffin pan.

5 Transfer the muffin pan to the oven, and bake for about 10 minutes, or until a toothpick inserted into a muffin comes out clean. Remove from the oven.

6 Let the muffins cool in the pan before removing them.

Storage: Store, covered, on the counter for about 3 days or in the refrigerator for up to 1 week.

Tip: You can easily make oat flour by processing rolled oats in a blender or food processor.

Hooray for Hummus Dip

PREP TIME: 10 to 15 minutes
DAIRY-FREE · **GLUTEN-FREE** · **NUT-FREE** · **VEGAN** · **VEGETARIAN**

Dips are the best! They offer a fun way to get kids interested in eating things they may not normally be into. Hummus is easy, delicious, healthy, and fun to scoop veggies in, and can be popular for snacking. This Middle Eastern side dish is packed with nutrients, and contains a good amount of plant protein, too. Hooray for hummus! MAKES 3 TO 4 CUPS

⅓ cup roasted tahini (sesame paste)

½ cup extra-virgin olive oil, plus more for garnish

1 tablespoon minced garlic, plus more for garnish

2 ½ (15-ounce) cans chickpeas, drained and rinsed

¼ cup fresh lemon juice, or to taste

½ cup filtered water

Sprinkle of paprika, for garnish

Carrot sticks, sliced cucumber, or crackers, for serving

Storage: Keep in a glass jar in the refrigerator for up to 5 days.

Tip: At the store, tahini is normally found by the nut butters, even though sesame is a seed.

1   Put the tahini, olive oil, garlic, chickpeas, lemon juice, and water in a food processor or blender. Pulse until smooth. Add more lemon juice to taste. Transfer to a bowl.

2   Garnish with olive oil, paprika, and garlic.

3   Serve with carrot sticks, cucumber slices, or crackers.

Roasted Cauliflower with Peanut Dip

PREP TIME: 15 minutes **COOK TIME:** 25 to 30 minutes
FREEZER-FRIENDLY · **DAIRY-FREE OPTION** · **GLUTEN-FREE OPTION** ·
VEGAN OPTION · **VEGETARIAN**

This family side is served with a fun peanut butter dip, which offers exposure
to the common allergen, peanuts. Dips and sauces make foods more enticing
for kids to try, as they can dunk vegetables or other foods into them. SERVES 4

FOR THE CAULIFLOWER:

2 heads of cauliflower, cut into florets

½ cup avocado oil or ghee

2 teaspoons smoked or plain paprika

1 teaspoon garlic powder

Pinch of freshly ground black pepper

FOR THE PEANUT DIP:

¼ cup warm filtered water

¼ cup plus 2 tablespoons creamy peanut butter

2 tablespoons rice wine vinegar

2 tablespoons fresh lime juice

2 teaspoons minced fresh ginger

1 teaspoon low-sodium soy sauce

1 teaspoon maple syrup or honey (only use
honey if over 12 months old)

TO MAKE THE CAULIFLOWER:

1   Preheat the oven to 425°F.

2   In a large bowl, toss together the cauliflower, avocado oil, paprika, garlic powder,
and pepper. Transfer to a baking sheet.

3   Transfer the baking sheet to the oven,
and roast for 25 to 30 minutes, or until
the cauliflower is soft and golden. Remove
from the oven.

TO MAKE THE PEANUT DIP:

1   While the cauliflower is cooking, in a glass
jar, combine the water, peanut butter,
vinegar, lime juice, ginger, soy sauce,
and maple syrup. Seal the lid and shake
vigorously.

2   Serve alongside the cauliflower as a dip
or drizzle.

Storage: Keep the cauliflower and dip in
separate airtight glass containers in the
refrigerator for up to 3 days.

Tip: You can substitute any nut or seed
butter here to avoid allergen exposure.
Note that soy sauce does contain gluten,
so if this is something you are avoiding for
your child, opt for a gluten-free alternative
such as tamari, or coconut aminos.

Sweet Potato Crackers

PREP TIME: 15 to 20 minutes, plus 10 minutes to chill until firm **COOK TIME:** 30 minutes

DAIRY-FREE · **GLUTEN-FREE** · **NUT-FREE** · **VEGAN** · **VEGETARIAN**

Crackers are a favorite kids' snack, but most store-bought crackers are filled with ingredients that don't support health or growth in any way. This recipe is a wonderful alternative. These homemade crackers are so easy to make and are insanely delicious. They're crunchy, savory, and easy to munch on. You might want to double the recipe, so you can enjoy them, too. **MAKES ABOUT 3 DOZEN**

8 TO 12 MONTHS

1 cup mashed cooked sweet potato

1 ½ cups oat flour

2 teaspoons fresh rosemary, minced

½ teaspoon garlic powder

¼ cup coconut oil, melted

1 Preheat the oven to 350°F. Line a 9 x 13-inch baking sheet with parchment paper.

2 In a medium bowl, combine the sweet potato, oat flour, rosemary, garlic powder, and coconut oil. Stir until a dough forms. Transfer to the prepared baking sheet, and place another sheet of parchment paper on top. Refrigerate for 5 to 10 minutes, or until firmed up.

3 Using a rolling pin, roll the dough into a thin layer, about ⅛ inch thick. The thinner the dough, the crispier the cracker.

4 Carefully remove the top layer of parchment paper. Using a pizza cutter, cut the dough into 1-inch squares.

5 Transfer the baking sheet to the oven, and bake for 15 minutes. Remove from the oven. Flip the crackers individually. Return the baking sheet to the oven, and bake for 15 minutes, or until the crackers are dry and crisp. Remove from the oven.

Storage: Keep in an airtight glass container at room temperature for up to 5 days.

Tip: If you don't have a rolling pin, you can use a canned good, water bottle, or tall drinking glass. If you don't have parchment paper, you can grease the baking sheet very well with coconut oil. Instead of the top layer of parchment paper, you can use plastic wrap with a rolling pin instead.

Sweet Potato Balls

PREP TIME: 15 minutes, plus 1 hour to chill

DAIRY-FREE · **GLUTEN-FREE** · **NUT-FREE** · **VEGETARIAN** · **VEGAN**

These little balls provide an easy alternative to the popular cereals for practicing the pincer grasp. The combination of healthy fats and a complex carb make them a good choice for both busy babies and breastfeeding parents. I love recipes that serve all ages as a quick snack! You can even make extra if you have an outing planned during the week, to avoid the temptation to buy something of lesser quality at the store in a pinch. **MAKES 12 TO 15 TEASPOON-SIZE BALLS**

1 cup mashed cooked sweet potato

3 tablespoons coconut oil

¼ teaspoon ground ginger

In a small bowl, mix together the sweet potato, coconut oil, and ginger until smooth. Refrigerate for 1 hour, or until cold. Then roll into teaspoon-size balls.

Storage: Keep in an airtight glass container in the refrigerator for up to 5 days.

Tip: You can use ghee or grass-fed butter if you are comfortable with dairy.

Pork Sausage Patties

PREP TIME: 15 to 20 minutes

COOK TIME: 10 minutes

GLUTEN-FREE · **NUT-FREE**

Homemade sausage patties like these are great for closer to 12 months or once dairy has been introduced. Patties are easy for little ones to hold on to, so they can self-feed. **MAKES 10 TO 12 PATTIES**

1 pound 80-percent-lean ground pork sausage

1 large egg

¼ cup cornstarch

¼ teaspoon paprika (optional)

½ cup grated raw cheese

¼ to ½ teaspoon dried sage

Coconut oil, for frying

1   In a large bowl, with clean hands, mix together the pork, egg, cornstarch, paprika (if using), cheese, and sage until well mixed. Form into 2-inch-wide, ½-inch-thick patties.

2   In a large skillet, heat a thin layer of coconut oil over medium-high heat.

3   Add the patties and cook, turning once, for 3 to 5 minutes on each side, or until cooked through. Remove from the heat.

Storage: Keep in an airtight glass container in the refrigerator for up to 3 days.

FINGER FOODS

Italian Cloud Bread

PREP TIME: 15 to 20 minutes **COOK TIME:** 15 minutes
GLUTEN-FREE · **NUT-FREE** · **VEGETARIAN**

These little flat rolls are easy to make and even easier for little hands to eat!
Serve these with Veggie Marinara (page 160) or other marinara sauce. You
can also use these rolls in place of sandwich bread for grilled cheese, as mini
pizza crusts, or topped with hummus or pâté. **MAKES ABOUT 12 ROLLS**

4 large eggs, separated

¼ teaspoon aluminum-free baking powder

½ teaspoon onion powder

½ teaspoon garlic powder

¼ teaspoon kosher salt

¾ teaspoon dried oregano

¼ cup cream cheese

3 tablespoons coconut oil

1   Preheat the oven to 325°F. Line a baking
sheet with parchment paper.

2   In a large bowl, combine the egg whites,
baking powder, onion powder, garlic
powder, salt, and oregano. Beat until firm
peaks form. This can take 4 to 5 minutes
depending on your equipment (by hand,
with a hand mixer, or a stand mixer).

3   In a medium bowl, combine the egg
yolks, cream cheese, and coconut oil. Mix
until smooth.

4   Carefully fold the egg yolk mixture into
the egg whites, maintaining the fluffi-
ness of the egg white mixture as much as
possible.

5   Using a large spoon, immediately spoon
about ⅓-cup portions of batter onto the
prepared baking sheet, forming 12 rolls.

6   Transfer the baking sheet to the oven
and bake for 15 minutes.

7   Let cool and serve.

Storage: Keep in an airtight glass container in the refrigerator for up to 2 to
3 days. To reheat, place in a toaster for
1 minute or warm in a skillet.

Tip: If the rolls end up running into
each other, making one big sheet of thin
bread, just use a pizza cutter to cut into
1 x 4-inch sticks and serve as dippers.

8 TO 12 MONTHS

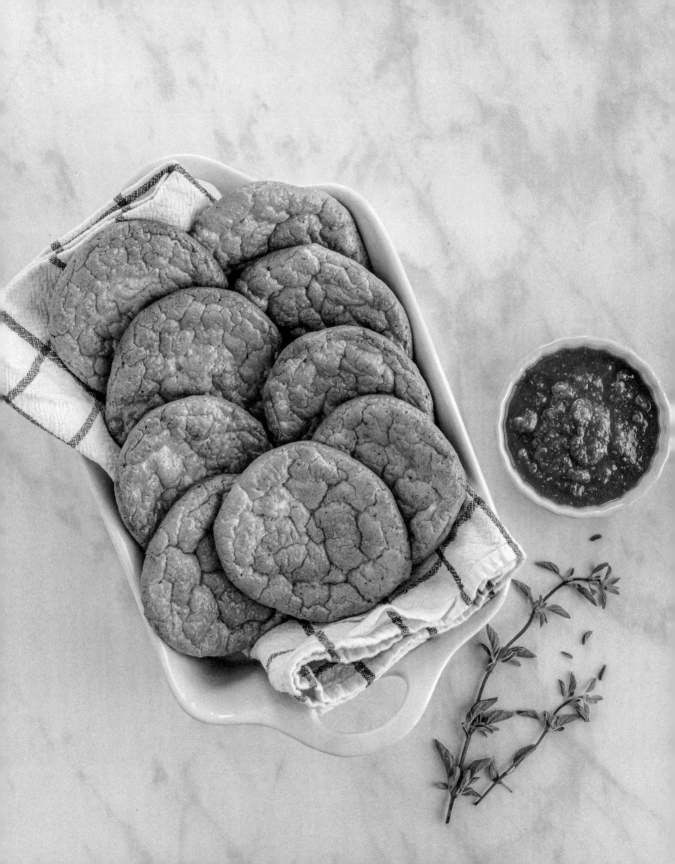

Chicken and Black Bean Quesadilla

PREP TIME: 5 minutes **COOK TIME:** 5 minutes
GLUTEN-FREE • **NUT-FREE** • **VEGETARIAN**

These yummy, cheesy quesadillas deliver a healthy, well-rounded meal
in one dish. Using sprouted corn tortillas can be a healthy alternative for
the popular white tortillas. If you can't find them, plain corn tortillas are
a good option, but wait to serve them until after 12 months, since it is a
grain. **SERVES 1 TO 2**

1 tablespoon grass-fed butter or coconut oil

2 sprouted corn tortillas

2 tablespoons finely diced cooked chicken

2 tablespoons black beans

¼ cup grated raw cheese

1 In a cast-iron skillet, melt the butter over
medium-low heat.

2 Put 1 tortilla in the skillet. Top with
the chicken and beans, followed by the
cheese. Place the second tortilla on top.
Cook for 2 minutes on each side, or until
the cheese has melted. Remove from
the heat.

3 Using a pizza cutter, cut into 4 or more
pieces, and let cool for 1 to 2 minutes
before serving.

Storage: Keep in an airtight glass container in the refrigerator for up to 2 to
3 days. The quesadillas taste best when
eaten within the first day or two.

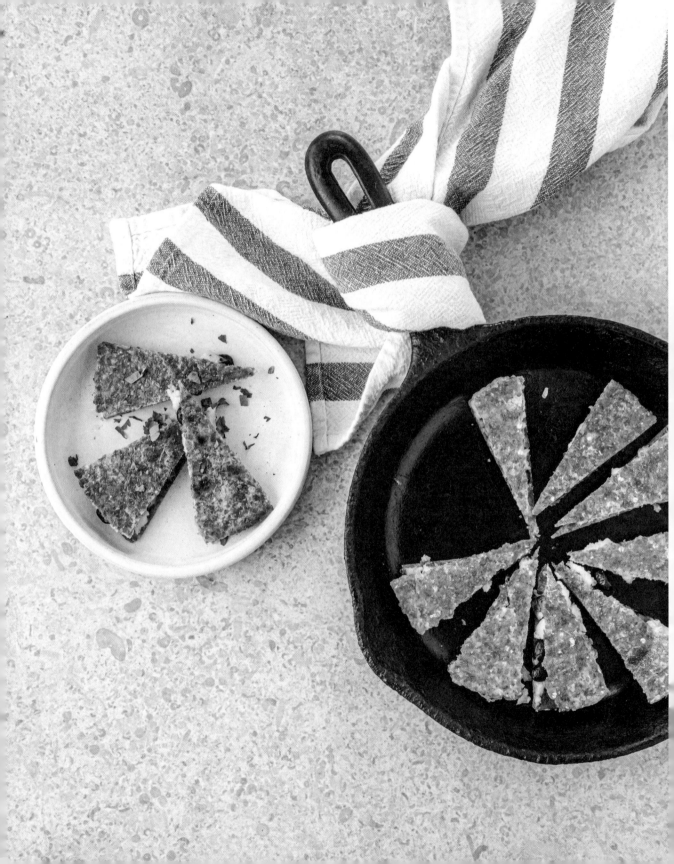

Mushroom and Black Olive Pizza

PREP TIME: 15 to 20 minutes **COOK TIME:** 35 to 45 minutes
GLUTEN-FREE • **NUT-FREE** • **VEGETARIAN**

Pizza is one of my favorite ways to involve kids in the kitchen. They decide which ingredients to use and pile toppings on. They are more into eating something when they've helped prepare it, so grab them and make it a pizza night for the family! **MAKES 1 REGULAR PIZZA OR 2 PERSONAL PIZZAS**

8 TO 12 MONTHS

FOR THE CRUST:

1 cup coconut flour

1 cup arrowroot powder

1 teaspoon kosher salt

1 teaspoon onion powder

1 teaspoon garlic powder

3 large egg yolks

1 cup coconut milk

½ cup coconut oil, warmed

FOR THE PIZZA:

½ cup marinara sauce

1 teaspoon Italian seasoning

½ cup mushrooms, sliced

½ cup black olives, sliced

1 cup shredded mozzarella cheese

TO MAKE THE CRUST.

1   Preheat the oven to 400°F. Line a baking sheet with parchment paper.

2   In a large bowl, mix together the coconut flour, arrowroot powder, salt, onion powder, and garlic powder.

3   In another bowl, mix together the egg yolks, coconut milk, and coconut oil.

4   Add the wet ingredients to the dry ingredients. Whisk to form a smooth dough without lumps. Set aside for 5 minutes to firm up.

5   Spread the dough out to ¼-inch thickness on the prepared baking sheet. Transfer the baking sheet to the oven, and bake for 25 to 30 minutes, or until golden brown underneath. If you want it a bit more crunchy, bake longer. Remove from the oven, leaving the oven on.

TO MAKE THE PIZZA:

1　In a medium bowl, mix together the marinara sauce and Italian seasoning. Spread the marinara sauce over the crust.

2　Add the mushrooms, olives, and cheese. Return the baking sheet to the oven, and bake for 10 to 12 minutes, or until the cheese has melted. Remove from the oven.

Storage: Keep in an airtight glass container in the refrigerator (if there is any left!) for up to 3 days.

Tip: It's best to buy a block of cheese and grate it yourself because pre-shredded cheese contains anticaking agents. Use jarred marinara sauce as pizza sauce and get either the garlic or basil flavor.

Veggie Marinara

PREP TIME: 15 to 20 minutes **COOK TIME:** 10 to 15 minutes
FREEZER-FRIENDLY · **DAIRY-FREE** · **GLUTEN-FREE** · **NUT-FREE** · **VEGAN** · **VEGETARIAN**

Although I am a big fan of introducing vegetables in a formal way, there's nothing wrong with disguising them in other foods to enhance a meal. This sauce is perfect for dipping or for pasta. It's packed with veggies, but if you're craving a meaty sauce, you can also add cooked ground meat. **MAKES 8 TO 10 CUPS**

3 tablespoons olive oil or avocado oil

3 bell peppers, cored and chopped

3 zucchini, chopped

3 yellow squash, chopped

1 (8-ounce) bag of spinach

2 (20-ounce) jars marinara sauce

1 In a large pot, heat the oil over medium heat.

2 Add the peppers, zucchini, and squash. Sauté for about 10 minutes, or until very tender.

3 Add the spinach and cook for 1 to 2 minutes. Remove from the heat. Transfer to a blender.

4 Add the marinara sauce. Blend on high speed for 45 to 60 seconds, or until smooth.

Storage: Once cooled, divide the marinara into large glass jars, leaving 1 inch at the top, and refrigerate for 3 days or freeze for up to 3 months.

8 TO 12 MONTHS

All-Organic Baby Food Cookbook

Healthy Smash Cake

PREP TIME: 10 to 15 minutes **COOK TIME:** 40 to 45 minutes
GLUTEN-FREE · **NUT-FREE** · **VEGETARIAN**

Just because you've decided to hold off on sugar and grains doesn't mean you and your baby have to miss out on a first birthday cake! Coconut flour can be dry, so there are seven (!) eggs in this recipe. A luscious banana and cream cheese frosting further adds moist deliciousness. This treat will surely be something to smash and enjoy without leaving them feeling crazed and then exhausted from a sugar crash. **MAKES 1 BIRTHDAY CAKE (WITHOUT A SUGAR CRASH)**

FOR THE CAKE:

2 to 3 tablespoons coconut oil, for greasing

¾ cup coconut flour

½ cup arrowroot powder

¼ cup shredded, unsweetened coconut

¼ teaspoon kosher salt

½ teaspoon aluminum-free baking soda

½ teaspoon ground cinnamon (optional)

⅔ cup coconut oil or ghee, melted

⅓ cup maple syrup

7 large eggs

2 tablespoons alcohol-free vanilla extract

¼ cup canned coconut cream

FOR THE FROSTING:

1 (8-ounce) package cream cheese, at room temperature

½ cup (1 stick) grass-fed, unsalted butter, at room temperature

1 medium banana, ripe and with spots

TO MAKE THE CAKE:

1   Preheat the oven to 325°F. Grease 2 cake pans.

2   In a large bowl, stir together the coconut flour, arrowroot powder, coconut, salt, baking soda, and cinnamon (if using).

3   In another bowl, mix together the coconut oil, maple syrup, eggs, vanilla, and coconut cream. ➤➤

4   Add the wet ingredients to the dry ingre-
    dients, and mix well to incorporate. Pour
    into the prepared pans.

5   Transfer the pans to the oven, and bake
    for 40 to 45 minutes, or until a toothpick
    inserted into the center comes out clean.
    Remove from the oven. Let cool fully
    before stacking and frosting.

TO MAKE THE FROSTING:

1   In a blender or using a hand mixer,
    blend the cream cheese, butter, and
    banana well.

2   Spread evenly over the cakes.

    Storage: Keep in an airtight glass con-
    tainer in the refrigerator (if there is any
    left!) for up to 3 days or freeze for up to
    3 months.

INTRODUCING MILK AT 12 MONTHS

If you're nursing at 12 months, there is no need to introduce cow's milk as a regular addition to the diet. Mother's milk contains richer fat content, necessary for your toddler's growing brain. Breast milk also contains more nutritional properties than cow's milk. Instead, focus on calcium and fat by offering a wide range of healthy fats (yogurt, oily fish, cheese, avocado, nut butters, butter, and coconut oil) to your baby. Cow's milk is just a convenient way to get in a combination of protein, fat, calcium and vitamin D, but it's not the only source. With my oldest, I transitioned her to goat's milk when I stopped nursing her around 17 months, and I also introduced her to cow's milk soon after. The choice is personal, and there is no right or wrong, as long as you wait until after 12 months of age.

Raw milk is controversial, but from a trusted, clean source, you are in good hands. If you want to transition your little one to cow's milk that is pasteurized, I recommend one with a local, low-heat pasteurization method such as vat- or batch-pasteurized milk. Whole organic cow's milk is the next best option, and you can do your own research on this (see Resources, page 234). There is nothing wrong with giving non-dairy milk, but it does not offer as much nutritional value and can contain additives like carrageenan or thickeners. If you go with non-dairy milk, be sure to read labels or make your own.

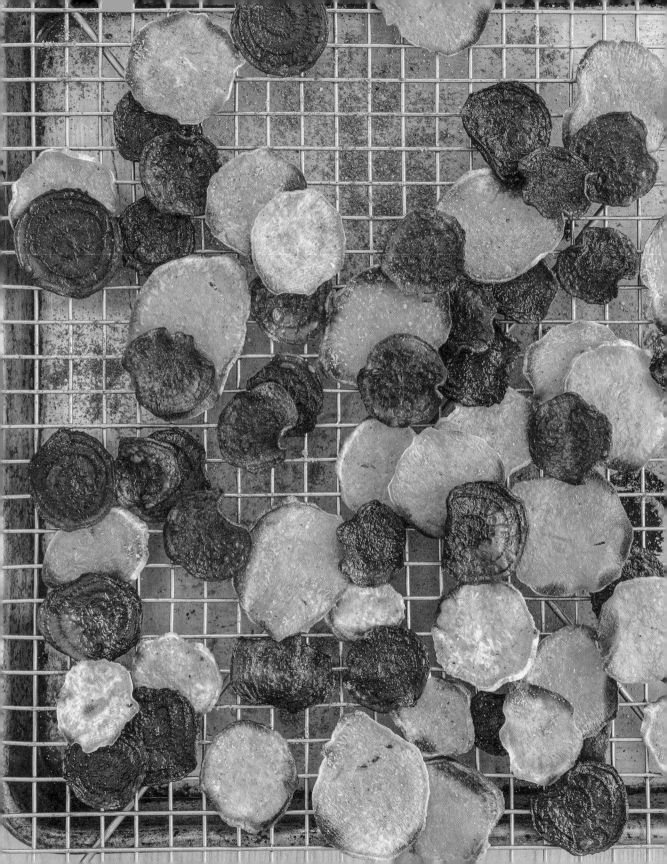

Eight

Toddler and Family Breakfasts & Snacks

12 TO 18 MONTHS+

The breakfast and snack recipes in this chapter are intended for the whole family to enjoy. Your busy toddler still may not eat a lot of food, but rather they may "graze," or eat a little bit throughout the day. You'll never want to force a child to eat at a meal time; rather, you'll want to listen to their body when they are hungry. Now's the time to begin conversations around "listening to your body" for hunger or thirst and also reading their body language when they become disinterested. A toddler who is done eating may not be able to tell you they are done, but by throwing their plate on the ground, they are indeed done and no longer interested in food at that time! Try to stay calm when this happens, knowing it is all part of building a positive relationship with food and a sense of some control over what and how much they choose to eat.

You may also notice your toddler gets "hangry"—angry because they're hungry or their blood sugar is getting low—and once they eat, they're suddenly cheerful. It may take reminding yourself that it isn't anger for anger's sake; they may be hungry but either don't realize it or don't know how to express it. Babies and toddlers cannot communicate, "Hey, I am hungry!" with their words. Mood swings in toddlers and young children are almost always related to one of three needs: a re-connection with a caregiver, food or drink, or sleep.

WHAT TO EXPECT

By this age, your children are mostly eating foods with "big people" textures, with caution toward choking hazards, such as slicing or serving them a certain way, and supervising specific foods (for example, berries, soft breads, cherry tomatoes, nuts, grapes, chunks of food, popcorn, and raw vegetables). Continue to offer spoons and forks, but don't necessarily expect them to be used. These months are more about practicing, but feeling free to use their hands.

How Much to Feed

¼ to 1 cup of food per meal, following your little one's lead and remembering that this changes during growth spurts, illness, and teething.

When to Feed

About 3 meals and 2 to 3 snacks a day. Some parents like to offer a snack-grazing atmosphere, so their child can choose when to eat, while others like to establish a mealtime routine.

What to Drink

Breast milk, formula, milk, or water are the only appropriate drinks to offer your baby at this age. There is no hard-and-fast rule to continue breastfeeding or wean; it is simply a decision for you and your baby. Some toddlers at 12 to 18 months begin on another form of milk, such as goat, cow, or other alternatives (see Introducing Milk at 12 Months, page 163).

First-Time Parent Tip

Around 12 months, I introduced a "help me to help myself" idea. I cleared out a kitchen drawer for my toddler to place their bowls, utensils, and plates as well as a low shelf in the pantry for their snacks for the day (bananas, avocados, and homemade crackers). I loved seeing my child's face when I showed them the new setup. I remember watching them happily grab a bowl and ask for help with a snack. This system encourages independence and helps us parents out, too, by allowing them to communicate their needs to us.

Spinach and Cheese Egg Scramble with Avocado

PREP TIME: 5 minutes **COOK TIME:** 5 minutes
GLUTEN-FREE • **NUT-FREE** • **VEGETARIAN**

This protein-packed scramble is the perfectly balanced breakfast, and colorful to boot. Spinach and avocado provide necessary greens and healthy fats for growing little ones and nourish the busy parent, too. To add even more color (and vitamin C), toss in some finely diced red bell pepper. **SERVES 2**

3 large eggs

¼ cup milk of choice

¼ cup fresh spinach, chopped

3 tablespoons shredded cheese

½ tablespoon grass-fed, unsalted butter, plus more for greasing the skillet

½ ripe avocado, pitted, peeled, and sliced

Sea salt and freshly ground black pepper to taste

1 In a medium bowl, whisk together the eggs and milk.

2 Stir in the spinach and cheese.

3 In a small, greased skillet, melt the butter over high heat.

4 Once the butter begins to brown, add the egg mixture. Cook undisturbed for 30 to 60 seconds, or until the edges solidify. Reduce the heat to very low. Using a fork, bring the cooked edges in toward the center while tilting the pan so the raw egg from the center runs to the edges. Cook undisturbed for 30 to 60 seconds, then scramble. Remove from the heat.

5 Add the avocado, season with salt and pepper to taste, and serve warm.

Storage: Keep in an airtight glass container in the refrigerator for up to 1 day.

Tip: An alternate super smooth option is to combine 3 raw eggs with 1 cup raw spinach in a blender. Blend on high speed until smooth. Scramble the green eggs in the skillet with cheese and a dash of salt and pepper.

Mom's Hash Brown and Sausage Casserole

PREP TIME: 5 to 10 minutes **COOK TIME:** 45 to 55 minutes
GLUTEN-FREE · **NUT-FREE**

This recipe was our Sunday morning breakfast my mom used to make when I was growing up. She made it a little different each time based on what ingredients we had, but this version was the one I remember most. It's hearty and filling, setting the family up for all the day's adventures. **SERVES 8**

10 large eggs

2 ¾ cups milk of choice

2 teaspoons kosher salt, plus more for seasoning

¼ teaspoon freshly ground black pepper, plus more for seasoning

½ teaspoon garlic powder

½ teaspoon onion powder

½ red bell pepper, cored and diced

1 (30-ounce) package of frozen shredded hash browns

2 cups shredded Cheddar cheese

8 sausage patties, cooked

1   Preheat the oven to 350°F.

2   In a large bowl, whisk together the eggs, milk, salt, pepper, garlic powder, and onion powder.

3   Mix in the bell pepper, hash browns, and cheese. Transfer to a 9 x 13-inch baking dish.

4   Place the sausage patties on top, pressing them down a bit.

5   Transfer the baking dish to the oven, and bake for 45 to 55 minutes, or until the egg in the middle of the casserole springs back when poked. Remove from the oven. Season with salt and pepper to taste.

Storage: Keep, covered, in the refrigerator for up to 5 days.

Tip: If you use cow's milk, this casserole will be fluffy, but if you decide to use non-dairy milk, consider adding 2 extra eggs.

Great-Grandmother's Biscuits

PREP TIME: 10 to 15 minutes **COOK TIME:** 10 to 15 minutes
NUT-FREE · **VEGETARIAN**

I don't believe there are "bad foods." I do believe we nourish our body best by eating whole foods, but not all ingredients can be tolerated by all bodies. This recipe is great for when the body is calling for regular, old-fashioned biscuits. My great-grandmother made them best, and I'm happy to share her recipe. I recommend serving these with room-temperature grass-fed butter mixed with sorghum or honey (if baby is over 12 months old). Delicious! **MAKES ABOUT 10 BISCUITS**

2 cups all-purpose flour, plus more for dusting

4 teaspoons aluminum-free baking powder

½ teaspoon kosher salt

½ cup (1 stick) grass-fed, unsalted butter, cold

⅔ cup cold milk

1   Preheat the oven to 450°F.

2   Sift the flour and baking powder into a bowl. Add the salt.

3   Cut the butter into the flour with a fork until it resembles course meal or crumbs Do not overwork it.

4   Add the milk, and stir it in gently until everything starts to stick together.

5   Dust a clean work surface with flour. Turn the dough out. Flatten and fold it 12 times, then roll the dough out to about ½ inch thick.

6   Using the top of a drinking glass, cut out biscuits from the dough. Transfer to a baking sheet.

7   Transfer the baking sheet to the oven. For small biscuits, bake for 10 to 12 minutes. For medium biscuits, bake for 12 to 14 minutes. Remove from the oven.

Storage: Keep in an airtight glass container on the counter for up to 3 days.

Overnight Oats

PREP TIME: 5 minutes, plus at least 12 hours to soak

DAIRY-FREE OPTION · **GLUTEN-FREE** · **VEGETARIAN** · **VEGAN OPTION** ·

Because we're busy parents, we understand how rushed mornings can feel trying to get everyone (including yourself) fed. This recipe can be made the night before and basically does the "cooking" for you by soaking. It's great fuel for a toddler on the go, a nursing mother (it boosts milk supply), or anyone who wants to make mornings simpler. It can be eaten cold or warmed the next day. **MAKES ABOUT 2 CUPS**

1 cup rolled oats

1 tablespoon apple cider vinegar

Pinch of kosher salt

Warm filtered water

3 tablespoons grass-fed, unsalted butter (optional)

2 teaspoons coconut oil

Large dollop of almond butter or peanut butter

2 tablespoons maple syrup or honey (if baby is over 12 months old)

Fresh fruit or berries, for topping

1   Put the oats, vinegar, and salt in a glass container.

2   Add enough warm water to cover, and leave at least an inch of water over the oats. Cover, and let sit at room temperature for 12 to 24 hours.

3   In the morning, warm the oats (if desired), and mix in the butter (if using), coconut oil, almond butter, and maple syrup. Top with berries or fresh fruit.

Storage: Keep in an airtight glass container on the counter for up to 3 days.

Tip: For an adult's bowl, you can mix in a scoop of collagen, which adds protein and, for moms, is helpful with birth recovery.

Blender Oat Pancakes

PREP TIME: 10 minutes **COOK TIME:** 10 to 20 minutes
FREEZER-FRIENDLY · **GLUTEN-FREE** · **NUT-FREE** · **VEGAN** · **VEGETARIAN**

Perfect for an adult or busy toddler. I make this recipe in bulk a couple times a month, refrigerate for the week, and freeze the rest. These pancakes warm nicely in a toaster straight from the refrigerator or freezer. Note that once the collagen is added, the batter gets thicker. It is perfectly fine, just use a smaller scoop of the mix, and cook a little longer (2 to 3 minutes on each side). You can also omit the collagen powder, but I like the added 20 grams of protein per scoop! **MAKES ABOUT 8 PANCAKES**

12 TO 18 MONTHS+

1 ⅓ cups milk of choice

1 tablespoon apple cider vinegar

1 ½ tablespoons olive oil or avocado oil

1 ½ tablespoons alcohol-free vanilla extract

2 cups rolled oats or oat flour

½ to 1 scoop collagen powder (optional)

2 teaspoons aluminum-free baking powder

¼ teaspoon baking soda

⅛ teaspoon kosher salt

1 ½ teaspoon grass-fed, unsalted butter

Toppings of choice, such as maple syrup, grass-fed butter, nut butter, hemp seeds, fruit, honey (if baby is over 12 months old)

1 In a blender, combine the milk, vinegar, oil, vanilla, oats, collagen powder (if using), baking powder, baking soda, and salt. Pulse for about 45 seconds, or until well blended.

2 In a medium skillet, melt the butter over medium heat.

3 Add about ¼ cup batter per pancake. Cook for 1 to 3 minutes on each side.

4 Remove from the heat and serve with toppings of your choice.

Storage: Once cooled, keep in an airtight glass container in the refrigerator for up to 5 days or in the freezer for up to 3 months.

Blueberry and Almond Smoothie

PREP TIME: 5 minutes

FREEZER-FRIENDLY · **DAIRY-FREE OPTION** · **GLUTEN-FREE** · **VEGETARIAN**

Nothing is as easy and versatile as a morning concoction of blended fruit, veggies, and proteins to kick-start your day, nor as convenient to take with you on the run. This creamy, blue smoothie is a quick breakfast with added protein and good fats. We rarely have leftover smoothies, but when we do, we pour them into ice pop molds for a frozen treat. You can also add a handful of leafy greens for extra nutrition. **MAKES ABOUT 2 CUPS**

1 fresh or frozen banana (fresh for a thinner consistency, frozen for thicker)

1 cup frozen blueberries, plus more for serving

2 tablespoons raw almonds

¾ cup milk of choice

1 tablespoon flax meal

Handful of ice

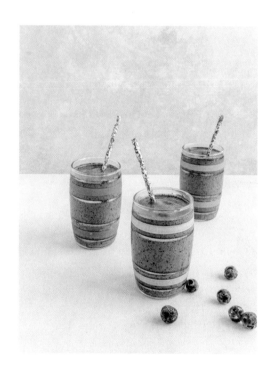

1 In a blender, combine the banana, blueberries, almonds, milk, flax meal, and ice. Blend for about 1 minute on high speed, or until smooth.

2 Serve in a glass, topped with more frozen blueberries.

   Storage: Keep in an airtight glass container in the refrigerator for up to 2 days.

   Tip: You could use any milk here, such as almond, coconut, oat, cow's, cashew, etc.

Pumpkin and Banana Smoothie

PREP TIME: 5 minutes

FREEZER-FRIENDLY · **DAIRY-FREE OPTION** · **GLUTEN-FREE** · **NUT-FREE** · **VEGETARIAN**

Smoothies are a great use for overripe bananas—just peel, chop, and freeze until ready to use. This warm flavor combo is wrapped up in a nice cool treat. Have a smoothie for breakfast or a snack. This recipe makes enough for you to share with your little one. **MAKES ABOUT 3 CUPS**

12 TO 18 MONTHS+

2 bananas, peeled, cut into chunks, and frozen

¾ cup pumpkin purée

2 to 3 tablespoons maple syrup or honey (if baby is over 12 months old)

1 teaspoon pumpkin pie spice

½ teaspoon ground cinnamon, plus more for topping

1 cup milk of choice

Handful of ice

1 In a blender, combine the bananas, pumpkin, maple syrup, pumpkin pie spice, cinnamon, milk, and ice. Blend for about 1 minute, or until smooth.

2 Serve in a glass, topped with more cinnamon.

Storage: Keep in an airtight glass container in the refrigerator for up to 2 days.

Tip: You could use any milk here, such as almond, coconut, oat, cow's, cashew, etc. Freeze leftover smoothie in an ice pop mold for a no-waste, fun treat.

Overnight Oatmeal Bake

PREP TIME: 10 minutes **COOK TIME:** 40 minutes
DAIRY-FREE OPTION · GLUTEN-FREE · NUT-FREE · VEGETARIAN

This blueberry oatmeal bake can be prepped the night before and left to soak, which enhances digestion, then baked the next morning. Or you can bake it right away. It's a special, hearty dish that makes breakfast easy all week long, whether you're home or on the go. **MAKES 24 BARS**

½ cup (1 stick) grass-fed, unsalted butter or coconut oil, melted, plus more for greasing

4 large eggs

1 cup maple syrup

2 teaspoons aluminum-free baking powder

½ teaspoon kosher salt

1 tablespoon ground cinnamon

2 tablespoons alcohol-free vanilla extract

2 cups milk of choice

6 cups quick oats

2 cups fresh blueberries

1   Preheat the oven to 350°F. Grease a 9 x 13-inch baking dish.

2   In a large bowl, whisk the eggs.

3   Add the maple syrup, baking powder, salt, cinnamon, and vanilla. Mix until smooth.

4   Add the milk and butter. Mix thoroughly.

5   Add the oats, stirring to combine.

6   Fold in the blueberries.

7   Spread the mixture into the prepared baking dish, smoothing it flat with a spatula.

8   Transfer the baking dish to the oven. Bake for 40 minutes, or until set. Remove from the oven. Once cool, cut into squares.

Storage: Keep in an airtight glass container at room temperature for up to 3 days.

Tip: You could substitute any berry here, like blackberry, raspberry, or strawberry.

Chia Seed Mousse

PREP TIME: 5 minutes, plus overnight to set

DAIRY-FREE · **GLUTEN-FREE** · **NUT-FREE OPTION** · **VEGAN OPTION** · **VEGETARIAN**

This 5-minute recipe can be added to squeeze pouches (yes, you can buy empty squeeze pouches and make your own!), served as a quick breakfast or snack, or added on top of fruit as a sweet treat. Chia is a complete protein packed with calcium, high in antioxidants (even more than blueberries), and full of omega-3s. **MAKES 3 TO 4 CUPS**

1 (15-ounce) can full-fat coconut milk

¼ cup black chia seeds

¼ teaspoon ground cinnamon

2 tablespoons maple syrup or honey (if baby is over 12 months old)

2 teaspoons alcohol-free vanilla extract

¼ cup unsweetened coconut flakes (optional)

¼ cup cocoa powder (optional)

A few tablespoons nut butter (optional)

Berries, fresh fruit, or Soaked Granola (page 189), for topping (optional)

1 Put the coconut milk, chia seeds, cinnamon, maple syrup, and vanilla in a medium bowl. Whisk well to combine so it gels evenly.

2 Stir in the coconut flakes (if using), cocoa powder (if using), and nut butter (if using). Pour into a glass jar, and refrigerate overnight. Serve with your favorite toppings (if using).

Storage: Keep in a glass jar in the refrigerator for up to 3 days.

Tip: The texture is like mousse. If you want something a little more like a pudding or yogurt, use coconut milk from a carton, not from a can.

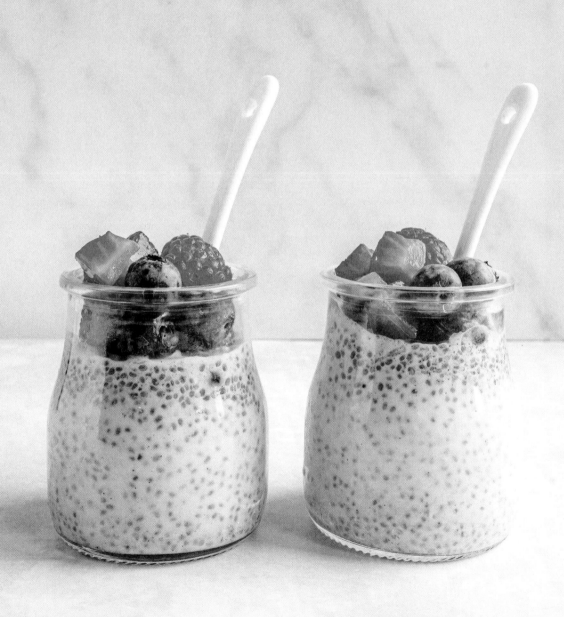

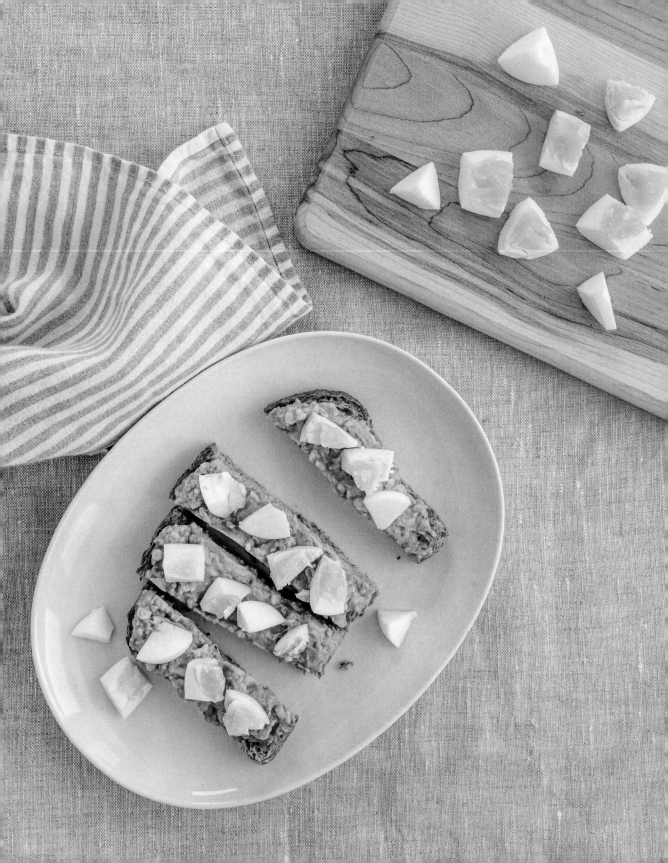

Avocado Toast Strips

PREP TIME: 5 to 10 minutes

DAIRY-FREE • **NUT-FREE** • **VEGETARIAN**

Avocado smeared on toast is a delicious creamy-crispy combination. Add some eggs and seasonings, and you've got a well-rounded, satiating breakfast. These toast strips are brain-boosting, thanks to avocado and hemp, and make a great snack or meal on the go. **SERVES 1 TO 2**

¼ to ½ ripe avocado, pitted and peeled

A few shakes of garlic powder

A few shakes of onion powder

1 slice sprouted grain or sourdough bread, lightly toasted

1 large egg, soft-boiled for 7 minutes, peeled, and sliced

2 teaspoons hemp seeds (optional)

Kosher salt and freshly ground black pepper to taste

1   Put the avocado in a small bowl, and lightly mash with a fork.

2   Add the garlic powder and onion powder. Spread on the bread.

3   Add the egg and hemp seeds (if using). Season with salt and pepper to taste.

4   Cut the avocado toast into 1-inch strips.

Storage: Keep the avocado mixture in an airtight glass container in the refrigerator for up to 3 days.

Tip: A sweet alternative to avocado is plain yogurt or nut butter with honey (if baby is over 12 months old). Omit the egg and seasonings, and add granola or extra hemp for a crunchy treat.

Yummy Gummies

PREP TIME: 10 minutes, plus 10 minutes to set **COOK TIME:** 1 minute
DAIRY-FREE • **GLUTEN-FREE** • **NUT-FREE**

Littles love gummies, but store-bought varieties are filled with sugar and artificial ingredients. These juicy, healthy snacks are designed for babies closer to 12 months of age, when they have a few more teeth. Always offer gummies with observation, since they could pose a choking risk. This treat also serves as a fantastic source of gelatin, outside of bone broth. MAKES

8 LARGE OR 16 TO 24 SMALL GUMMIES

12 TO 18 MONTHS+

Coconut oil, for greasing

½ cup **fresh juice of choice not from concentrate, such as orange, apple, or berry**

8 teaspoons **unflavored gelatin powder**

1 Grease a small baking dish.

2 Pour the juice into a small saucepan, and sprinkle the gelatin on the top. Let sit for 10 minutes. Then cook over low heat, stirring continuously for 1 minute or so, or until the gelatin has dissolved. The mixture will be thick like syrup. Remove from the heat. Immediately pour into the baking dish. Freeze for 10 minutes, or until set. Cut into shapes.

Storage: Keep in a glass jar in the refrigerator for up to 3 days.

Tip: You can make these into immunity or vitamin gummies by adding vitamin C powder, elderberry, or probiotics. Just stir them in with the juice before adding the gelatin. You can also make these in silicone molds. Kids love their fun shapes.

Blueberry Fruit Leather

PREP TIME: 5 minutes, plus 1 to 2 hours to thaw **COOK TIME:** 2 ¼ hours
DAIRY-FREE · **GLUTEN-FREE** · **NUT-FREE** · **VEGETARIAN**

I remember eating conventional fruit leathers as an after-school snack way too often as a kid. Too bad many of them are full of high fructose corn syrup, red dye number 40, and artificial flavors. Here's a recreation of those nostalgic childhood times, with a healthy spin your kids (and you!) will love. MAKES 10 TO 12 STRIPS

3 cups frozen blueberries, thawed for 1 to 2 hours

1 apple, cored and chopped

2 tablespoons maple syrup or honey (if baby is over 12 months old)

1 Preheat the oven to 170°F or the lowest possible temperature. Line a baking sheet with nonstick aluminum foil or a silicone baking mat.

2 In a blender, combine the blueberries, apple, and maple syrup. Blend on high speed until smooth, scraping down the sides as needed. Transfer to a saucepan. Cook over medium heat for 12 to 13 minutes, stirring occasionally, or until bubbling constantly. Remove from the heat. Pour onto the prepared baking sheet. Tap the sheet several times to pop bubbles and distribute evenly.

3 Transfer the baking sheet to the oven, and bake for 2 hours, checking every 25 to 30 minutes, or until the fruit leather is slightly dry to the touch and doesn't come off on your fingers.

4 Cut into strips, rolling them up. Or place strips onto parchment paper cut to size, and roll.

Storage: Keep in an airtight glass container at room temperature for about 1 month or freeze for up to 6 months.

Creamy Fudge Pops

PREP TIME: 5 minutes, plus at least 4 hours to freeze

FREEZER-FRIENDLY · **DAIRY-FREE** · **GLUTEN-FREE** · **NUT-FREE** · **VEGAN** · **VEGETARIAN**

Fudge pops should be part of every kid's (and parent's!) life. After all, what's summertime without them—they're the perfect ending to a day in the sun. Now you can make a healthy, creamy version at home that offers healthy fats and antioxidant-rich cocoa. **MAKES 6 FUDGE POPS**

12 TO 18 MONTHS+

1 (15-ounce) can full-fat coconut milk

½ cup unsweetened, dark cocoa powder

⅓ cup maple syrup

1 tablespoon alcohol-free vanilla extract

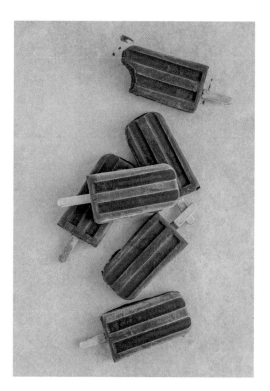

1   In a blender, combine the coconut milk, cocoa powder, maple syrup, and vanilla.

2   Blend on high speed until smooth. Pour into ice pop molds or paper cups (inserted with small ice pop sticks).

3   Freeze for at least 4 hours or up to overnight.

Storage: Keep in an airtight glass container in the freezer for up to 3 months.

Tip: Try using cacao, a less processed form of cocoa, if it's available.

Oatmeal, Chocolate Chip, and Pecan Cookies

PREP TIME: 15 to 20 minutes **COOK TIME:** 10 to 15 minutes

FREEZER-FRIENDLY · **DAIRY-FREE OPTION** · **GLUTEN-FREE** · **VEGETARIAN**

A cross between a hearty oatmeal cookie and a chocolate chip cookie, these little treats are the best combination of sweet, healthy, and filling. The almond flour and oats provide protein and fiber, while the good fats make it a not-so-guilty pleasure to enjoy with your family. **MAKES 30 TO 36 COOKIES**

1 ½ cups quick or rolled oats

1 cup almond flour

½ teaspoon kosher salt

½ teaspoon baking soda

½ cup maple syrup or honey (if baby is over 12 months old)

½ cup (1 stick) grass-fed, unsalted butter, at room temperature or melted coconut oil

2 large eggs

1 tablespoon alcohol-free vanilla extract

1 cup dark chocolate chips

1 cup pecan pieces

1 Preheat the oven to 350°F. Line a baking sheet with parchment paper.

2 In a medium bowl, whisk together the oats, flour, salt, and baking soda.

3 Add the maple syrup, butter, eggs, and vanilla. Stir well to combine.

4 Fold in the chocolate chips and pecans.

5 Drop about 2 tablespoons of batter about 1 inch apart onto the prepared baking sheet.

6 Transfer the baking sheet to the oven, and bake for 10 to 11 minutes, or until the edges start to turn golden. Remove from the oven. These cookies are a little fragile when they are warm, so let them cool for several minutes before removing them so they don't break.

Storage: Keep in an airtight glass container at room temperature for up to 5 days.

Blueberry Mini Muffins

PREP TIME: 20 minutes **COOK TIME:** 15 to 20 minutes
FREEZER-FRIENDLY · **DAIRY-FREE** · **GLUTEN-FREE** · **VEGETARIAN**

Mini muffins are somehow more fun than big muffins. They're also easy for little hands to grip. The added flax meal gives your family a boost of omegas from a plant-based source. You can alternatively make these without berries, adding the same amount of nuts or dried fruit. **MAKES 24 TO 30 MINI MUFFINS**

¼ cup coconut oil, melted, plus more for greasing (optional)

1 ¼ cups almond flour

2 ½ tablespoons coconut flour

¼ teaspoon kosher salt

1 teaspoon ground cinnamon

1 tablespoon flax meal

½ teaspoon baking soda

¼ cup maple syrup or honey (if baby is over 12 months old)

2 large eggs

1 tablespoon alcohol-free vanilla extract

1 cup fresh blueberries

1   Preheat the oven to 350°F. Grease a mini muffin pan (if desired), or place paper liners in the pan.

2   In a medium bowl, whisk together the almond flour, coconut flour, salt, cinnamon, flax meal, and baking soda.

3   In another bowl using a handheld mixer (or using a stand mixer), beat the melted coconut oil and maple syrup on medium-low speed until thick.

4   With the mixer running, add the eggs. Beat until combined.

5   Reduce the speed to low. Add the dry ingredients and mix until thick.

6   Stir in the vanilla.

7   Mix in the blueberries. Scoop small scoops of batter into the prepared muffin pan.

8   Transfer the muffin pan to the oven, and bake for 16 to 18 minutes, or until a toothpick inserted into a muffin comes out clean. Remove from the oven.

Storage: These muffins keep on the counter, covered, for a couple days or in the freezer for up to 3 months.

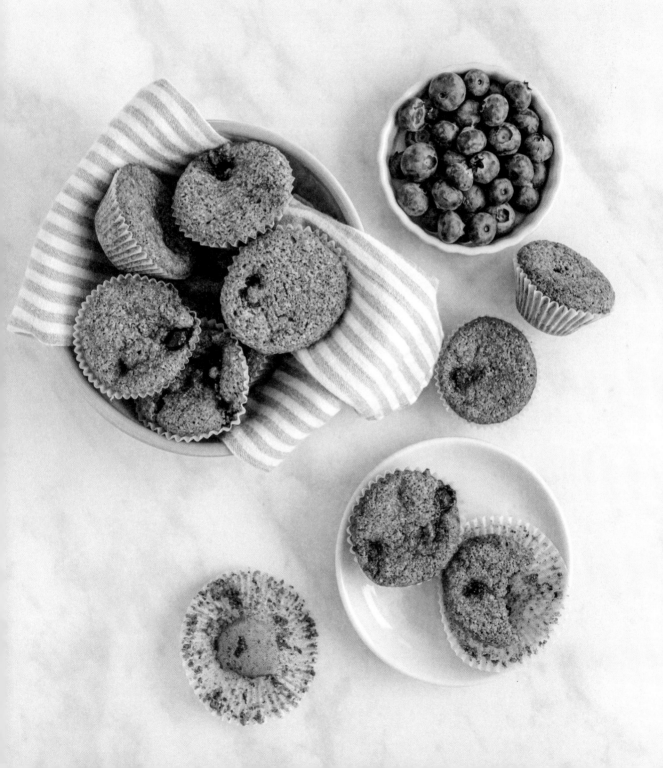

Guacamole

PREP TIME: 10 to 15 minutes
DAIRY-FREE · **GLUTEN-FREE** · **NUT-FREE** · **VEGAN** · **VEGETARIAN**

Guacamole, easy to make and loved by all, really spices up the superfood avocado. Serve alongside the Chicken and Black Bean Quesadilla (page 156), on top of the Black Bean Enchiladas with Spinach and Cheese (page 230), or even instead of the avocado on the Spinach and Cheese Egg Scramble (page 168). You can also try it right on toast! MAKES ABOUT 3 CUPS

12 TO 18 MONTHS+

3 ripe avocados, halved, pitted, and peeled

½ small red onion, diced

2 roma tomatoes, diced (optional)

3 tablespoons fresh cilantro, chopped

2 garlic cloves, minced, or 1 ½ teaspoons garlic powder

Juice of 1 lime

Kosher salt and freshly ground black pepper to taste

1   Put the avocados in a medium bowl, and mash with a fork.

2   Add the onion, tomatoes (if using), cilantro, garlic, and lime juice. Season with salt and pepper. Stir to combine.

Storage: Keep covered with plastic wrap in an airtight glass container in the refrigerator for 3 days.

Tip: Rolling a lime on the counter before cutting helps it release more juice.

Root Veggie Chips

PREP TIME: 10 to 15 minutes **COOK TIME:** 15 to 25 minutes
DAIRY-FREE · GLUTEN-FREE · NUT-FREE · VEGAN · VEGETARIAN

Colorful, crispy, root vegetable chips make a perfect snack or side to a nourishing meal. This is a good recipe to involve your little ones in the kitchen. Let them transfer the sliced veggies to a big bowl. These chips are great for older toddlers who can munch on something crunchy successfully. Always supervise littles when they are eating a chip-type snack because of the choking risk. To make thinly sliced chips of even thickness, use a mandoline. **MAKES ABOUT 3 CUPS**

3 tablespoons melted coconut oil, plus more for greasing

2 medium beets, peeled and cut into ¹⁄₁₆-inch-thick slices

2 medium sweet potatoes, peeled and cut into ¹⁄₁₆-inch-thick slices

½ teaspoon kosher salt

¾ teaspoon garlic powder

½ teaspoon paprika, ground cumin, or dried oregano (optional)

1 Preheat the oven to 375°F. Lightly grease 2 baking sheets.

2 Put the beets and sweet potatoes in separate bowls.

3 Divide the coconut oil, salt, garlic powder, and paprika (if using) evenly between the bowls. Toss to coat. Transfer the beets to one prepared baking sheet, and the sweet potatoes to the other. Spread them out in an even layer.

4 Transfer the baking sheets to the oven, and bake for 15 to 25 minutes, flipping halfway through, or until crispy and wrinkled, but not browned. Remove from the oven.

Storage: Keep in an airtight glass container at room temperature for up to 1 week.

Tip: You could use yucca, plantain, taro, white or yellow potato, or parsnips as alternatives.

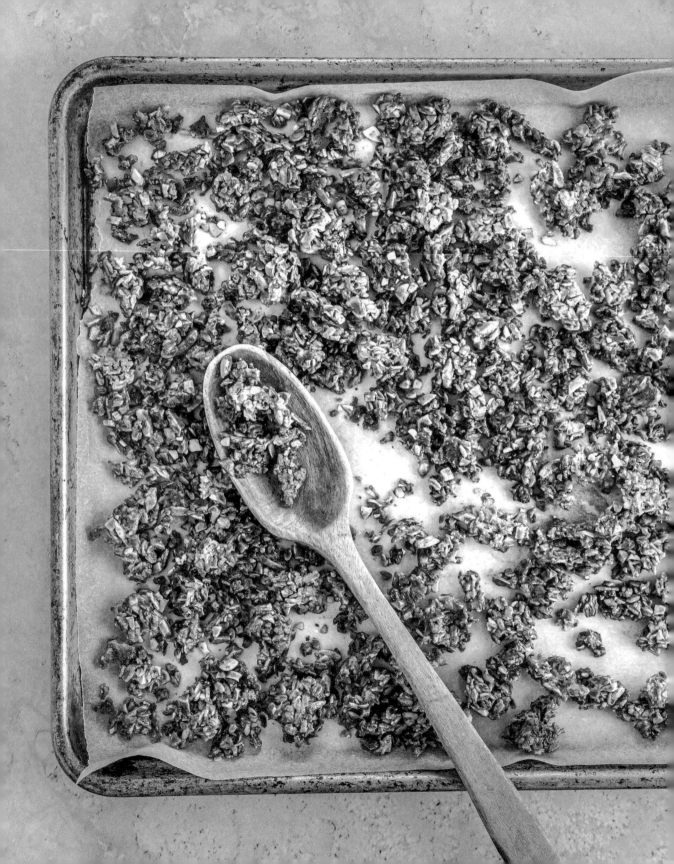

Soaked Granola

PREP TIME: 5 minutes, plus at least 8 hours to soak **COOK TIME:** 10 to 14 hours
DAIRY-FREE OPTION • **GLUTEN-FREE** • **VEGETARIAN**

Store-bought granola tends to have a lot of sugar and not-so-natural flavorings. This granola is made from ingredients you probably have in your kitchen and can be served as the perfect breakfast with yogurt, on-the-go snack, or smoothie topping. Soaking the oats allows the grain to be broken down, making the grain more easily digested and the nutrients more absorbable. Soaking the nuts begins the process of germination, which deactivates enzyme inhibitors, further unlocking their nutritional benefits. My introduction to healthful granola came when one of my first midwives brought me a big jar for boosting my milk supply when I was just a few days postpartum. **MAKES 7 CUPS**

4 cups rolled oats

Warm filtered water

½ cup whey (see page 135), apple cider vinegar, or fresh lemon juice

1 cup almonds (2 cups if omitting pepitas)

1 cup raw pepitas (optional)

½ cup coconut oil

2 tablespoons alcohol-free vanilla extract

½ cup maple syrup or raw honey (if baby is over 12 months old)

2 tablespoons ground cinnamon

½ teaspoon ground nutmeg

1. Put the oats in a large bowl, and cover with warm water.
2. Stir in the whey. Cover, and let sit for 8 hours or up to overnight.
3. Put the almonds and pepitas (if using) in a separate bowl. Cover with warm water. Let sit for 8 hours or up to overnight.
4. The next morning, preheat the oven to 120°F or the lowest possible temperature. Line 2 baking sheets with parchment paper.
5. Drain the oats, almonds, and pepitas.
6. Finely chop the almonds and pepitas. Mix into the oats. Spread out evenly onto the prepared baking sheets. ➔

7   Transfer the baking sheets to the oven, leaving the door slightly ajar to allow moisture to escape.

8   Dehydrate for 8 to 10 hours, or until dry, checking and turning the mixture with a spatula every few hours to make sure it dries evenly. Remove from the oven, leaving the oven on.

9   In a pot, heat the coconut oil, vanilla, and maple syrup over low heat until the oil has melted.

10   Stir in the cinnamon and nutmeg. Remove from the heat. Pour over the oats, stirring to coat evenly.

11   Return the baking sheets to the oven, and bake for 2 to 4 hours, or until crisp. Remove from the oven. Let cool.

Storage: Keep in an airtight container in a cool, dry place for up to 1 month.

Tip: You could use another nut in place of almonds, like walnuts or pecans. If you have a convection setting on your oven, use it! The air flow will speed up your drying process.

Sprouted Nut Butter Dippers

PREP TIME: 10 minutes, plus overnight to soak **COOK TIME:** 12 to 24 hours
DAIRY-FREE • **GLUTEN-FREE** • **VEGETARIAN**

I love to have nut butter on hand for busy toddlers. It's a great addition to any meal or smoothie, and it works well for dipping our favorite fruits or veggies. Just a reminder that soaking and dehydrating nuts reduces the phytic acid content, allowing them to be more easily digested (see page 36). The protein content per tablespoon of this recipe really attracts me to this snack idea, since my kids are often eating just a bite or two of something before they are off to play. **MAKES ABOUT 1 ¾ CUPS**

2 cups raw nuts (see Tip)

1 tablespoon plus ½ teaspoon kosher salt

Filtered water

1 tablespoon almond, coconut, or walnut oil

1 tablespoon maple syrup or honey (if baby is over 12 months old)

Dippers, such as sliced apple, carrot, cucumber, or celery

1 In a large bowl, combine the nuts and 1 tablespoon of salt. Cover with water by at least 1 inch. Let soak overnight.

2 The next morning, preheat the oven to 300°F.

3 Drain and rinse the nuts. Spread out evenly onto a baking sheet.

4 Transfer the baking sheet to the oven, and bake for 1 hour. Turn off the oven, stir the mixture, and leave it in the oven to dry for 12 hours or overnight. Make sure they are completely dry, then remove from the oven. Transfer to a blender.

5 Add the remaining ½ teaspoon of salt. Blend on high speed until the nuts turn into powder, and continue blending for another 30 seconds or so.

6 Add the oil and maple syrup. Blend to your desired consistency, scraping down the sides with a spatula as needed. Serve with dippers.

Storage: Keep in an airtight glass jar in the refrigerator for up to several weeks.

Tip: If using cashews, soak for only 6 hours and bake at 200°F instead for 6 hours.

Nut Butter Power Bites

PREP TIME: 5 minutes, plus 2 hours to freeze **COOK TIME:** 5 minutes
FREEZER-FRIENDLY · **DAIRY-FREE OPTION** · **GLUTEN-FREE** · **VEGETARIAN**

These treats double as both parent fuel and toddler fuel, their healthy fats
are brain-boosting, and they're so quick to whip up! Even though one of these
little bars seem small, the energy it delivers is huge. Perfect for a toddler on
the go or who's in a particularly active phase, and would rather be playing
than interacting with food for longer than a few minutes. My former boss and
midwife would also make these for the nurses to keep us going during long
births when we were up all night! **MAKES 16 TO 20 BARS**

12 TO 18 MONTHS+

1 ½ cups mix-ins of choice, such as hemp seeds,
dark chocolate chips, sliced almonds, other nuts
(optional)

2 cups peanut butter or any nut butter

2 cups coconut oil or 1 cup coconut oil plus 1 cup
(2 sticks) grass-fed, unsalted butter

½ cup maple syrup or honey (if baby is over
12 months old)

1   Put the mix-ins (if using) into an
8 x 8-inch baking dish.

2   Put the peanut butter, coconut oil, and
maple syrup in a saucepan. Cook over low
heat, whisking constantly to make sure
the mixture does not bubble and burn,
until combined. Remove from the heat.
Pour into the baking dish. Freeze for
2 hours. Cut into 1-inch blocks and serve.

Storage: Keep in an airtight glass container in the refrigerator for up to 7 days
or in the freezer for up to 3 months.

Tip: If making for children less than
12 months old, grind the nuts first, and
use maple syrup, not honey.

EASY TODDLER SNACKS

Prepackaged foods geared toward babies, toddlers, and kids are so tempting, but they usually contain additives like unhealthy oils or refined sugars. However, there happen to be some fresh and healthy store-bought "convenient" foods that make prep time minimal or non-existent. Following are some of my favorites:

- Full-fat cottage cheese with veggies, fruit, or homemade crackers
- For 21 months and up, raw carrots and cucumbers, quartered tomatoes, plain or in a salad
- Antibiotic- and nitrate-free turkey or chicken deli meat rollups with sliced or string cheese
- Nitrate-free pepperoni or salami rolls with cream cheese
- Dried seaweed sheets
- Dried fruit or dehydrated fruit (mango, raisins, or cherries; no sugar added)
- Hard-boiled eggs
- Clementine or mandarin oranges (a favorite for peeling and fine motor skill promotion)

- Trail mix (soaked nuts with dried fruits, a brain-boosting combo that doubles as both toddler fuel and parent brain food)
- Apples slices and nut butter mixed with maple syrup or honey (if baby is over 12 months old)
- Celery (12 months, sliced into thin half-moons; 2 years, matchsticks) and petite carrot sticks with hummus or nut butter
- Fresh fruit or berries
- Halved olives or fermented pickles

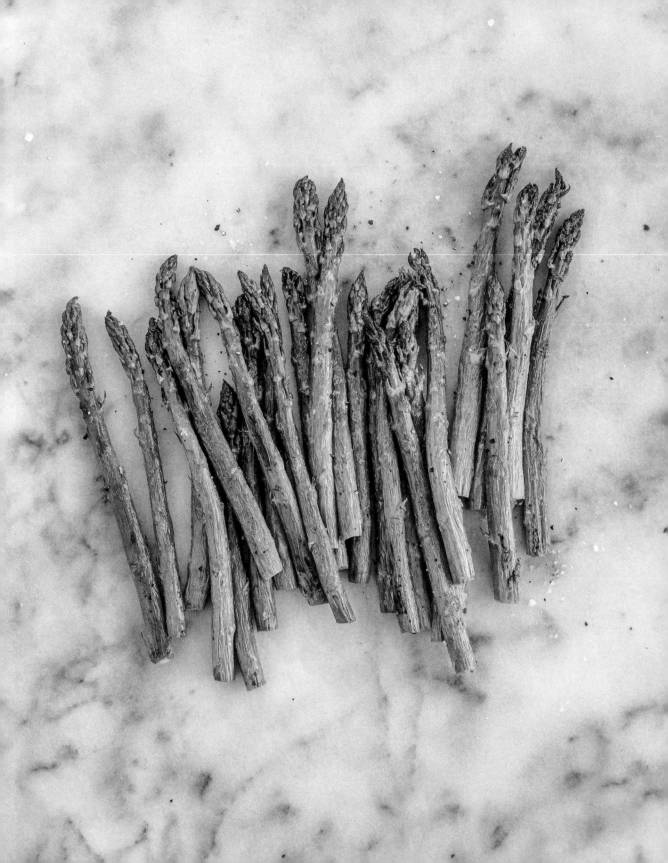

Nine

Toddler and Family Sides & Mains

12 TO 18+ MONTHS

In this chapter, you'll discover some main dishes and sides to enjoy together as a family. Involve your kids in food preparation and cooking to continue encouraging baby's healthy relationship with nourishing food. It may take twice as long to get a meal on the table, but it's a big part of life, and the more kids are exposed to these activities at a young age, the more it'll stick with them as they grow. This can be as simple as letting them transfer chopped vegetables into a big bowl or spread foods out on the baking sheet. My kids love to stir cookie batter with their own child-size spatulas. Kids who help prepare food are also more likely to try the foods they've helped make. You might be surprised by what they will taste-test while cooking; even things that they may have rejected in the past.

WHAT TO EXPECT

By this age, your children are mostly eating foods with "big-people" textures, with caution to choking hazards, slicing and serving them a certain way, and supervising specific foods (including berries, soft breads, cherry tomatoes, nuts, grapes, chunks of food, popcorn, and raw vegetables). Continue to offer spoons and forks, but don't necessarily expect them to be used. Utensils are still more for practicing, but toddlers should feel free to use their hands.

How Much to Feed
¼ to 1 cup of food per meal, following your little one's lead and knowing that this changes during growth spurts, illness, and teething.

When to Feed
About 3 meals and 2 to 3 snacks a day. Some parents like to offer a snack-grazing atmosphere, so their child can choose when to eat, while others like to establish a mealtime routine.

What to Drink
Breast milk, formula, milk, or water remain the only appropriate drinks to offer your baby at this age. There is no rule to continue breastfeeding or wean; it is simply a decision for you and your baby. As tempting as it is, don't offer juice or boxed "kid drinks." You can make your own fresh juice or homemade lemonade with honey as a seldom-offered special treat.

First-Time Parent Tip
It can be tempting, and I've been guilty of it, but resist the urge to use bribes or rewards during mealtime. Instead, teach kids that mealtime is mealtime, and while they should try a new food, they don't need to be rewarded or praised for it. Bribing teaches them to eat their "healthy meal" just so they can have a "treat." This tends to cement the idea that the meal is less desirable than the treat. When there is resistance to a new food, I find my children more interested in trying it once I reply to their "NO!" with "Okay, you don't have to try it. Only if you want to," Without any emotions on my end.

Loaded Summer Salad

PREP TIME: 20 to 25 minutes
DAIRY-FREE · **GLUTEN-FREE** · **NUT-FREE**

A summer favorite in our house: loaded salads. In what was kind of an accident, I combined what we had left over in the refrigerator with some fresh items from our garden, creating this perfect combo of proteins, greens, and vegetables for a sunny day. **SERVES 1 TO 2**

FOR THE BALSAMIC VINAIGRETTE:

½ cup olive oil

¼ cup balsamic vinegar

1 teaspoon maple syrup or honey (if baby is over 12 months old)

1 teaspoon Dijon mustard

1 garlic clove, minced

Kosher salt and freshly ground black pepper to taste

FOR THE SALAD:

1 ½ to 2 cups mixed greens

½ cup chopped cooked chicken

½ ripe avocado, pitted, peeled, and diced

1 small radish, thinly sliced

¼ orange bell pepper, cored and diced

1 soft-boiled egg, peeled and halved

¼ cup diced tomato

1 tablespoon toasted pumpkin seeds

1 tablespoon toasted sunflower seeds

TO MAKE THE BALSAMIC VINAIGRETTE:

1   In a glass jar, combine the olive oil, vinegar, maple syrup, mustard, and garlic.

2   Season with salt and pepper to taste. Seal the lid, and shake vigorously.

TO MAKE THE SALAD:

1   In a large bowl, combine the mixed greens, chicken, avocado, radish, bell pepper, egg, and tomato.

2   Add the vinaigrette, and toss to coat.

3   Sprinkle the pumpkin and sunflower seeds on top.

Storage: Dressing will keep in a sealed glass jar in the refrigerator for up to a week.

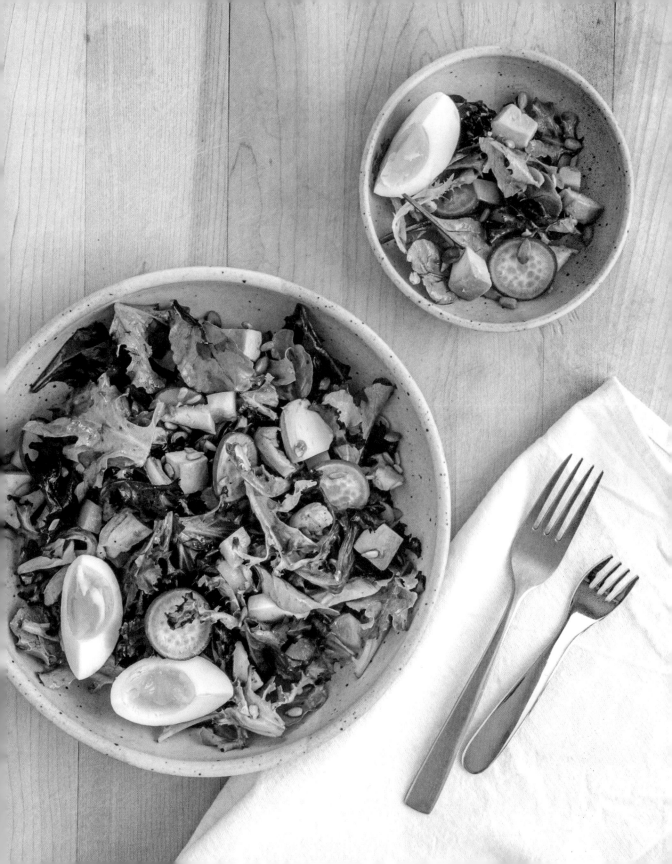

Eggcellent Egg Salad

PREP TIME: 25 minutes

GLUTEN-FREE · NUT-FREE · VEGETARIAN

This salad is a good way to mix up the versatile and powerful food—eggs. I like to serve this on sourdough toast, wrapped in butter lettuce, or scooped up with crackers. A lot of store-bought mayo is made with soy or canola oil, but this healthier homemade option is made with olive oil. **MAKES ABOUT 2 CUPS MAYONNAISE AND 1 ¾ CUPS EGG SALAD**

FOR THE MAYONNAISE:

1 cup sour cream or Greek yogurt

2 large egg yolks

¼ cup apple cider vinegar

1 tablespoon Dijon mustard

1 tablespoon maple syrup or honey (if baby is over 12 months old)

½ teaspoon kosher salt

¼ cup olive oil

FOR THE EGG SALAD:

5 large eggs, hard-boiled, peeled, and sliced

1 to 2 pickles, finely chopped

¼ cup homemade mayonnaise

1 teaspoon Dijon mustard

Kosher salt and freshly ground black pepper to taste

Fresh dill, for garnish (optional)

TO MAKE THE MAYONNAISE:

1   In a blender, combine the sour cream, egg yolks, vinegar, mustard, maple syrup, and salt. Blend for about 30 seconds.

2   With the blender running, slowly add the olive oil. Blend until the mixture thickens into mayonnaise. Pour into a glass jar with a lid. It will thicken more in the refrigerator.

TO MAKE THE EGG SALAD:

1   In a medium bowl, combine the eggs, pickles, mayonnaise, and mustard. Season with salt and pepper to taste. Mix well, and mash with a fork.

2   Garnish with dill (if using).

Storage: Keep the salad in an airtight glass container in the refrigerator for up to 3 days. The mayonnaise will keep for about 7 days.

Four-Bean Salad

PREP TIME: 15 to 20 minutes, plus up to 2 hours to soak the beans

DAIRY-FREE · GLUTEN-FREE · NUT-FREE · VEGAN · VEGETARIAN

Enjoy a rainbow of beans in this tasty and filling plant-based side. Although I normally recommend soaking dried beans, a quick canned bean salad is easy to prepare. This quick-soak method still involves soaking the beans for a few hours to break them down, but if you don't have time, feel free to skip this step. Make sure to grab BPA-free cans. **MAKES ABOUT 10 CUPS**

1 (15-ounce) can pinto beans, drained and rinsed

1 (15-ounce) can chickpeas, drained and rinsed

1 (15-ounce) can black beans, drained and rinsed

1 (15-ounce) can kidney beans, drained and rinsed

Filtered water

2 tablespoons apple cider vinegar

½ large red onion, diced

1 green bell pepper, cored and diced

1 red bell pepper, cored and diced

½ teaspoon kosher salt

½ teaspoon freshly ground black pepper

½ cup red wine vinegar

2 tablespoons maple syrup

¼ cup olive oil

1   In a large bowl, combine the pinto beans, chickpeas, black beans, and kidney beans. Cover with filtered water by 1 inch, and add the cider vinegar. Let soak for 1 to 2 hours, then drain. Rinse and dry the bowl.

2   In the same bowl, combine the beans, onion, green bell pepper, and red bell pepper.

3   In a small bowl, make the dressing. Whisk together the salt, pepper, red wine vinegar, and maple syrup. Slowly pour in the olive oil, whisking to combine.

4   Pour the dressing over the beans, and toss. Serve immediately, or for the flavor to develop, cover and refrigerate for at least 4 hours or up to overnight. Toss again before serving.

Storage: Keep in an airtight glass container in the refrigerator for up to 3 days.

Cucumber Salad with Dill Yogurt Dressing

PREP TIME: 5 minutes
GLUTEN-FREE · **NUT-FREE** · **VEGETARIAN**

This summery dish is perfect for a quick meal, side, or even a snack. Cucumbers are hydrating and refreshing, and they pair perfectly with the yogurt and dill. Try letting your little helper place all the cucumbers in a bowl after you cut them. **MAKES ABOUT 1 CUP**

½ cup plain Greek yogurt or sour cream

Juice of 1 lemon

½ teaspoon kosher salt

½ teaspoon freshly ground black pepper

2 tablespoons chopped fresh dill

2 medium cucumbers, thinly sliced

1   In a medium bowl, whisk together the yogurt, lemon juice, salt, pepper, and dill.

2   Add the cucumbers, and toss to combine.

Storage: Keep in an airtight glass container in the refrigerator for up to 1 day.

ABC Broccoli Slaw

PREP TIME: 20 minutes
GLUTEN-FREE

This slaw complements any meal, especially a family picnic. As your kids help throw the A=apple (or almond), B=bacon (or broccoli), and dried C=cranberries into the mix, they will also get a lesson in the alphabet. A lot of store-bought mayonnaise is made with soy or canola oil, which is why I use my homemade version made with olive oil instead. **MAKES ABOUT 6 CUPS**

½ cup homemade Mayonnaise (page 200)

½ tablespoon apple cider vinegar

2 tablespoons maple syrup

¼ teaspoon garlic powder

1 head of broccoli, finely chopped

¼ pound bacon, cooked and chopped

¼ cup dried cranberries

½ apple, cored and cut into ¼-inch dice

¼ cup sliced almonds

½ red onion, finely diced

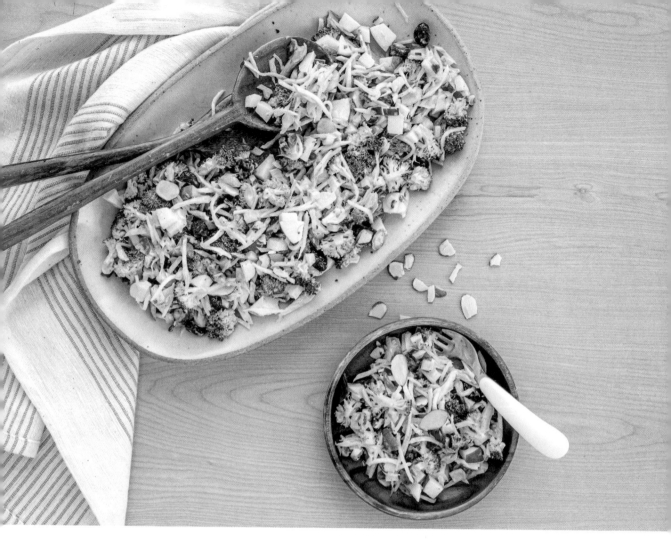

1 In a medium bowl, whisk together the mayonnaise, vinegar, maple syrup, and garlic powder.

2 Add the broccoli, bacon, cranberries, apple, almonds, and onion. Toss to combine. Serve immediately, or refrigerate for about 1 hour to let the flavors meld.

Storage: Keep in an airtight glass container in the refrigerator for up to 3 days.

Tip: Dried cherries or raisins are a good substitute for dried cranberries; pecans, walnuts, or sunflower seeds are a good substitute for sliced almonds.

Asparagus Rex

PREP TIME: 5 minutes **COOK TIME:** 15 minutes

DAIRY-FREE · **GLUTEN-FREE** · **NUT-FREE** · **VEGAN** · **VEGETARIAN**

Using fun language for foods is a sure way to get kids interested in trying a new (or not commonly offered) food. Asparagus Rex can be offered as dinosaur tails! Asparagus is on the Clean Fifteen list, so it's not as impacted by pesticides. Buying conventionally grown is usually okay, and it leaves more for your organic budget. **SERVES 4 TO 6**

1 to 2 pounds fresh asparagus, woody ends removed

1 to 3 tablespoons avocado oil

Kosher salt and freshly ground black pepper to taste

Tip: You could use melted ghee or coconut oil instead of avocado oil.

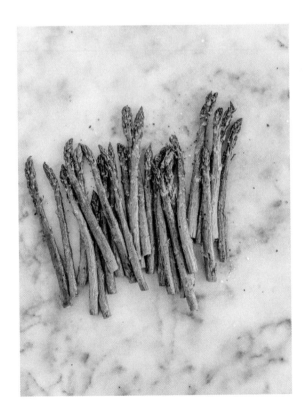

1   Preheat the oven to 450°F.

2   Put the asparagus on a baking sheet.

3   Drizzle the avocado oil on top. Season with salt and pepper to taste.

4   With clean hands, roll the asparagus around to coat evenly. Arrange into a single layer.

5   Transfer the baking sheet to the oven, and roast for about 15 minutes, turning halfway through. Remove from the oven.

Storage: Keep in an airtight glass container in the refrigerator for up to 4 days.

Sweet Potato Fries

PREP TIME: 10 to 15 minutes, plus 30 minutes to soak **COOK TIME:** 25 to 30 minutes

DAIRY-FREE OPTION · GLUTEN-FREE · NUT-FREE · VEGAN OPTION · VEGETARIAN

Fries are a good addition to almost any meal. They're well-liked by just about everyone, and they make terrific finger foods for little hands. Sweet potato fries are a great alternative to regular French fries, with long-lasting complex carbohydrates. They're also rich in beta-carotene, and best of all, fun to dip. **SERVES 4**

2 large or 4 small sweet potatoes, peeled and cut into ¼-inch-thick matchsticks

Cold filtered water

2 tablespoons avocado oil

2 tablespoons cornstarch

½ teaspoon garlic powder

½ teaspoon smoked paprika

Kosher salt and freshly ground pepper to taste

Sour cream, for dipping (optional)

1   Put the sweet potatoes in a large bowl of cold water, and soak for 30 minutes. Drain and pat dry. Wipe out the bowl. Return the sweet potatoes to the bowl.

2   Preheat the oven to 425°F. Line 2 baking sheets with parchment paper.

3   Add the avocado oil to the bowl, and toss to coat the sweet potatoes evenly.

4   In a small bowl, mix together the cornstarch, garlic powder, and smoked paprika. Sprinkle evenly over the sweet potatoes, and toss until evenly coated. Spread out evenly onto the prepared baking sheets, make sure the sweet potatoes don't overlap.

5   Transfer the baking sheet to the oven, and bake for 25 to 30 minutes, flipping halfway through, or until crispy and the tips have started to brown. Remove from the oven. Let cool. Season with salt and pepper to taste. Serve with sour cream (if using).

Storage: Keep in an airtight glass container in the refrigerator for up to 3 days.

SIDES

Cheesy Mashed Cauliflower

PREP TIME: 15 to 20 minutes **COOK TIME:** 20 minutes
GLUTEN-FREE · NUT-FREE OPTION · VEGETARIAN

Cauliflower has enjoyed a rise in popularity due to its versatility; it can be riced, roasted, and in this case, mashed. This easy alternative to mashed potatoes makes a perfect comfort side. You can easily omit the milk and cheese, and use a dairy-free milk for a similar creamy side. **MAKES ABOUT 4 CUPS**

12 TO 18+ MONTHS

Filtered water

1 head of cauliflower, stemmed and chopped

¼ cup whole milk or nut milk

2 tablespoons (¼ stick) grass-fed, unsalted butter or ghee

Kosher salt and freshly ground black pepper to taste

1 cup grated white Cheddar cheese

1 tablespoon chopped fresh chives

1   Bring a medium pot of water to a boil.

2   Add the cauliflower, and boil for 15 minutes, or until fork-tender. Drain and return it to the empty pot.

3   Add the milk and butter. Season with salt to taste. Cook over low heat, and mash until creamy. Season with pepper to taste.

4   Turn off the heat and quickly stir in the cheese and chives. Cover with a lid to melt the cheese.

Storage: Keep in an airtight glass container in the refrigerator for up to 3 days.

Tip: For a super-creamy texture, you could blend the cauliflower before adding the cheese.

Cranberry Pecan Chicken Salad

PREP TIME: 15 to 20 minutes
GLUTEN-FREE

Chicken salad has been making lunches and snacks easier for years. Think about it: It's great to make up a batch for the week, and enjoy as a quick snack or lunch on sourdough toast, wrapped in butter lettuce, or scooped up with crackers. No matter how you serve it, it's always good with ripe tomatoes, lettuce, or avocado. A lot of store-bought mayo is made with soy or canola oil. This uses my homemade version, made with olive oil instead. **SERVES 6**

2 cups chopped cooked chicken

2 celery stalks, chopped

¼ cup dried no-sugar-added cranberries

¼ cup pecans, chopped

¼ cup homemade Mayonnaise (page 200)

2 teaspoons Dijon mustard

Kosher salt and freshly ground black pepper to taste

In a large bowl, combine the chicken, celery, cranberries, pecans, mayonnaise, and mustard. Season with salt and pepper to taste. Mix well.

Storage: Keep the salad and mayonnaise in separate airtight glass containers in the refrigerator. The mayonnaise will keep for about 7 days and the salad for up to 3 days.

SIDES

Easy Fried Rice

PREP TIME: 10 minutes **COOK TIME:** 10 minutes
DAIRY-FREE · **GLUTEN-FREE OPTION** · **NUT-FREE** · **VEGETARIAN**

Using leftover rice for fried rice makes it fresh again, and its dry texture is ideal for blending with other ingredients. This recipe only takes about 20 minutes to whip up and is a perfect side for a roasted meat or fish. It's also a nice add-in to a lunch bowl with whatever meats, veggies, and sauce you have on hand. **MAKES ABOUT 6 CUPS**

12 TO 18+ MONTHS

1 tablespoon olive oil

1 teaspoon minced garlic

¼ large sweet Vidalia onion, chopped

1 cup frozen peas and carrots

3 cups cooked rice

2 large eggs

½ teaspoon sesame oil

3 tablespoons low-sodium soy sauce

1 bunch of scallions (green parts only), chopped (optional)

1 In a large skillet or wok, heat the olive oil over medium heat.

2 Add the garlic and onion. Cook, stirring continuously, for 2 to 3 minutes, or until the onion begins to soften.

3 Add the peas and carrots, and cook, stirring, for 1 to 2 minutes, or until the peas begin to thaw.

4 Raise the heat to medium-high. Add the cooked rice, and cook for 2 to 3 minutes.

5 Reduce the heat to medium-low. Make a space in the middle of the skillet by pushing the rice to the edge.

6 Crack the eggs into the empty space, and scramble. Cook for 1 to 2 minutes, or until set, then stir them into the rice mixture to combine. Remove from the heat.

7 Stir in the sesame oil, soy sauce, and scallions (if using).

Storage: Keep in an airtight glass container in the refrigerator for up to 4 days.

Tip: Soy sauce contains gluten, so if this is something you are avoiding for your child, opt for a gluten-free alternative such as coconut aminos or a gluten-free soy sauce.

Rainbow Spinach Salad

PREP TIME: 10 minutes
GLUTEN-FREE • **VEGETARIAN**

This immunity-packed salad is a perfect spring dish. With food of nearly every color, you really get a rainbow! The flavors of the goat cheese mixed with the freshly grated beet and pickled onion deliver a combination of tangy, creamy, and crispy. It's perfect for letting little ones choose what they want to try on top of a salad. **SERVES 2**

1 ½ to 2 cups fresh spinach

1 teaspoon sauerkraut

3 tablespoons raw baby beet, grated

1 large carrot, grated

1 tablespoon pickled red onion

Balsamic vinaigrette, for serving

Olive oil

Raw pecans and goat cheese crumbles, for toppings

1 In a large bowl, combine the spinach and top with the sauerkraut, beet, carrot, and pickled onion.

2 Drizzle with balsamic vinaigrette and olive oil.

3 Sprinkle the pecans and goat cheese on top.

Storage: Once combined, this salad should be enjoyed immediately. Keep ingredients stored separately in airtight glass containers in the refrigerator until ready to serve.

Tip: Make this an interactive salad, too. Ask your toddler to describe the flavors of some of the toppings (sweet, sour) and the texture (creamy, crunchy) to encourage fun sensory involvement.

Four-Bean Chili with Veggies

PREP TIME: 15 minutes **COOK TIME:** 25 to 30 minutes
FREEZER-FRIENDLY · **DAIRY-FREE** · **GLUTEN-FREE** · **NUT-FREE**

It's a bit longer on ingredients, but this hearty recipe is a staple in my house. I always double this recipe and freeze half. It makes a nice big pot for sharing or for enjoying a quick meal on a busy night, when the only work is pulling out a jar of chili and thawing it in the refrigerator overnight. **MAKES ABOUT 3 QUARTS**

1 tablespoon olive oil

1 small onion, diced

1 ½ teaspoons chopped garlic

1 ¼ quarts bone broth

2 to 3 carrots, chopped

1 celery stalk, chopped

1 sweet potato, diced

1 zucchini, diced

1 bell pepper, cored and chopped

1 ½ teaspoons kosher salt

1 teaspoon freshly ground black pepper

1 tablespoon chili powder

1 (15-ounce) can black beans, drained and rinsed

1 (15-ounce) can pinto beans, drained and rinsed

1 (15-ounce) can kidney beans, drained and rinsed

1 (15-ounce) can cannellini beans, drained and rinsed

1 In a large pot, heat the olive oil over medium-high heat.

2 Add the onion, and sauté for 2 to 3 minutes, or until beginning to soften.

3 Stir in the garlic, and sauté for 1 minute.

4 Add the broth, carrots, celery, sweet potato, zucchini, and bell pepper.

5 Stir in the salt, pepper, chili powder, black beans, pinto beans, kidney beans, and cannellini beans. Bring to a boil. Reduce the heat to a simmer, cover with a lid, and cook for 20 minutes. Remove from the heat.

Storage: Keep in an airtight glass container in the refrigerator for up to 4 days or freeze for up to 6 months.

Tip: For more probiotic power, you can garnish with avocado and top with kefir or sauerkraut.

12 TO 18+ MONTHS

One-Pot Hearty Winter Stew

PREP TIME: 20 minutes **COOK TIME:** 1 hour 45 minutes
FREEZER-FRIENDLY · **DAIRY-FREE** · **GLUTEN-FREE** · **NUT-FREE**

Full of meat, potatoes, veggies, noodles, and herbs, this recipe delivers the warmest bowl of comfort on a cold winter night. You can easily double the recipe to make a huge batch of stew, either for sharing or splitting in half to freeze some for a future meal. **MAKES 3 TO 4 QUARTS**

2 tablespoons olive oil

1 pound grass-fed beef chuck roast

½ pound grass-fed ground beef

1 to 2 chicken livers (optional)

1 ¼ teaspoons kosher salt

1 ½ teaspoons plus ¼ teaspoon freshly ground black pepper

1 ½ teaspoons plus ¼ teaspoon onion powder

1 ½ teaspoons plus ¼ teaspoon garlic powder

2 onions, chopped

2 carrots, chopped

1 ½ quarts beef bone broth

1 teaspoon dried sage

1 teaspoon dried oregano

1 (8-ounce) can green beans, drained and rinsed

1 potato, chopped

1 cup gluten-free macaroni pasta

1 In a large pot, heat the olive oil over high heat.

2 Add the beef chuck roast. Sear for 3 to 4 minutes on each side, or until browned on both sides. Transfer to a plate.

3 Reduce the heat to medium-high. Add the ground beef and liver (if using). Cook, breaking up the ground beef, for about 5 minutes, or until browned. Season with ¼ teaspoon of salt, ¼ teaspoon of pepper, ¼ teaspoon of onion powder, and ¼ teaspoon of garlic powder. Transfer to another plate.

4 Reduce the heat to medium. Add the onions and carrots. Cook for 8 to 10 minutes, or until soft. ➻

5   Add the broth, sage, oregano, remaining 1 teaspoon of salt, remaining 1 ½ teaspoons of pepper, remaining 1 ½ teaspoons of onion powder, and remaining 1 ½ teaspoons of garlic powder.

6   Add the chuck roast, green beans, and potato. Bring to a boil. Cover with a lid, reduce the heat to a simmer, and cook for 1 hour.

7   Add the ground beef, liver (if using), and pasta. Cook, uncovered, until the pasta is tender. Remove from the heat.

8   Spoon off the chuck roast and put pieces into bowls then top with soup, or carefully remove the chuck roast, and once it is cool enough to handle, cut into chunks, and return to the soup.

Storage: Store in an airtight glass container in the refrigerator for up to 4 days or in large quart jars in the freezer for up to 6 months. Leave 1 inch at the top for the stew to expand when it freezes.

Tip: Organ meat, such as liver, heart, or kidney, is a good a source of heme iron—try adding a few tablespoons to this recipe. You could opt for whole-wheat noodles if your baby is at least 18 months old and not sensitive to gluten.

One-Pot Chicken and Shrimp Gumbo

PREP TIME: 15 to 20 minutes **COOK TIME:** 45 to 50 minutes
FREEZER-FRIENDLY · **DAIRY-FREE OPTION** · **GLUTEN FREE OPTION** · **NUT-FREE**

A one-pot meal makes my night, like this quick, tasty gumbo to eat over the course of a few days. Toddlers often like things served separately, so you might offer the finished dish deconstructed so they can inspect any new foods. **MAKES 2 TO 3 QUARTS**

½ cup (1 stick) grass-fed, unsalted butter or olive oil

½ cup whole wheat-flour or oat flour

1 onion, diced

1 to 2 tablespoons minced garlic

1 red bell pepper, cored and diced

1 green bell pepper, cored and diced

2 celery stalks, chopped

2 teaspoons Cajun seasoning

2 bay leaves

3 ½ to 4 cups bone broth

1 pound andouille sausage, cut into 1-inch pieces

2 pounds boneless, skinless chicken thighs

¾ pound frozen okra

1 pound shrimp, peeled, deveined, and tails removed

1 In a large pot, melt the butter over medium heat.

2 Add the flour, and whisk continuously until it's the consistency and color of melted peanut butter.

3 Add the onion, garlic, red bell pepper, green bell pepper, celery, and Cajun seasoning. Cook for 3 to 5 minutes, or until the vegetables start to soften.

4 Add the bay leaves. Cook for 1 to 2 minutes.

5 Add the bone broth, sausage, chicken, and okra. Bring to a boil. Reduce the heat to a simmer, cover with a lid, and cook for 20 to 25 minutes.

6 Add the shrimp. Return to a simmer, and cook for about 5 minutes, or until pink.

7 Remove the chicken to a cutting board. Shred with 2 forks, return to the pot, and stir to combine. Remove from the heat. Discard the bay leaves. Serve in bowls.

Storage: Keep in an airtight glass container in the refrigerator for 3 to 4 days, or divide into glass jars after cooling and freeze for up to 6 months.

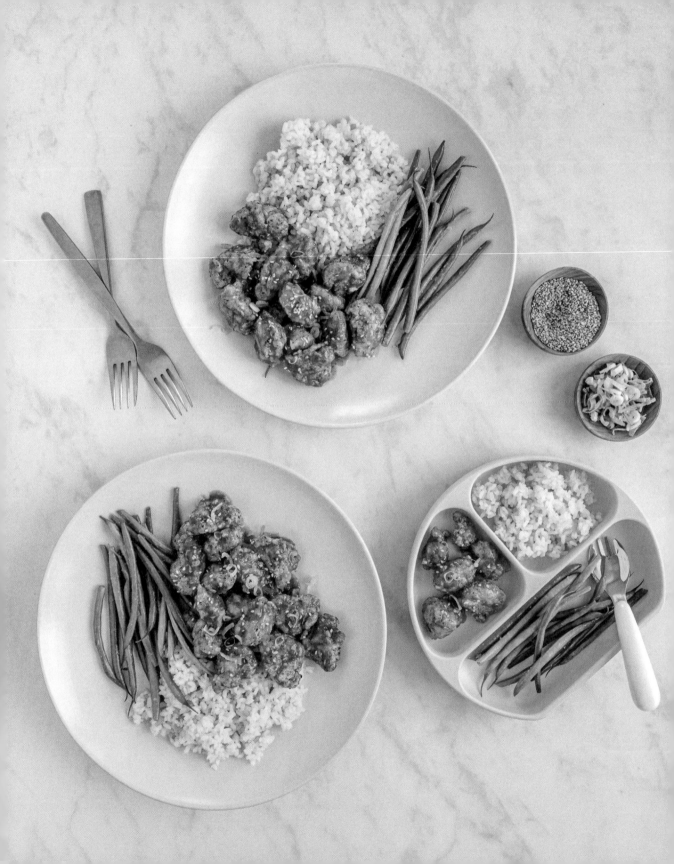

Mandarin Chicken with Garlic Green Beans

PREP TIME: 25 minutes **COOK TIME:** 30 minutes
FREEZER-FRIENDLY · **GLUTEN FREE OPTION**

Every kid (and parents, too) loves a bit of fried chicken every now and then. This chicken doesn't contain the bad stuff that "drive-thru" does, and is even more delicious! Pairing it with a side of green beans makes for a delicious meal you may even want to add to your weekly rotation. This dish is also perfect on its own or served over warm rice. **SERVES 6**

MAINS

FOR THE CHICKEN:

1 cup whole-wheat flour or almond flour

½ cup plus 2 tablespoons cornstarch

2 teaspoons kosher salt

2 teaspoons freshly ground black pepper

2 teaspoons garlic powder

2 large eggs

Filtered water

1 cup coconut oil

2 pounds boneless, skinless chicken thighs or breasts, cut into bite-size pieces

3 tablespoons cold filtered water, plus more as needed

Grated zest of 3 oranges

Juice of 3 oranges

2 tablespoons fresh lemon juice

¼ cup low-sodium soy sauce

1 tablespoon minced garlic

¼ cup maple syrup or honey (if baby is over 12 months old)

FOR THE GREEN BEANS:

1 pound green beans, trimmed

2 tablespoons (¼ stick) grass-fed, unsalted butter

½ teaspoon garlic powder

Kosher salt to taste

TO MAKE THE CHICKEN:

1 In a large bowl, stir together the flour, ½ cup of cornstarch, the salt, pepper, and garlic powder.

2 In a separate bowl, beat together the eggs and water.

3 In a large skillet, heat the coconut oil over medium heat. ➤➤

4   Once the oil is hot, dip the chicken into the egg mixture, then into the flour mixture. Drop into the oil, and cook undisturbed for 3 to 5 minutes on each side, or until cooked through. Remove from the heat.

5   In a small bowl, dissolve the remaining 2 tablespoons of cornstarch in the cold water. Whisk until combined.

6   To make the sauce, in a medium saucepan, stir together the orange zest and juice, lemon juice, soy sauce, garlic, and maple syrup. Bring to a simmer over medium-low heat, add the cornstarch slurry, and cook for.about 15 minutes, or until thickened to your desired consistency.

TO MAKE THE GREEN BEANS:

1   Meanwhile, set a steaming basket in a large saucepan, put in about 1 inch of water, and bring to a boil, making sure the water does not touch the bottom of the basket.

2   Put the green beans in the basket, tightly cover with a lid, and steam for about 7 minutes, or until tender. Remove from the heat. Transfer to a bowl.

3   Add the butter and garlic powder. Toss to distribute evenly. Season with salt to taste. Serve with the chicken. Pour the sauce over the chicken, and toss to coat evenly.

Storage: Keep in an airtight glass container in the refrigerator for up to 3 days.

Tip: To save time, make the sauce the night before and reheat before serving. You can also steam the green beans the night before as well. If desired, garnish with scallions and roasted sesame seeds. Soy sauce contains gluten, so if this is something you are avoiding for your child, opt for a gluten-free alternative such as tamari or coconut aminos.

One-Pan Roasted Salmon with Zucchini and Carrot Fries

PREP TIME: 15 to 20 minutes **COOK TIME:** 20 to 25 minutes
DAIRY-FREE · **GLUTEN-FREE** · **NUT-FREE**

Roasting is a wonderful cooking method that brings out the flavor and sweetness of foods, especially veggies. This colorful one-pan meal is a breeze to throw together. It lets you roast some vegetables and salmon and leaves just one pan to clean! SERVES 4

4 (4- to 6-ounce) wild-caught salmon fillets, pin bones removed

2 tablespoons maple syrup

2 to 3 tablespoons avocado oil or olive oil, plus more for drizzling

Kosher salt and freshly ground black pepper to taste

2 teaspoons garlic powder

4 large carrots, cut into matchsticks

1 large zucchini, cut into matchsticks

1 teaspoon paprika

1   Preheat the oven to 400°F.

2   Coat the salmon with the maple syrup and a drizzle of oil. Season with salt and pepper to taste and 1 teaspoon of garlic powder.

3   In a large bowl, combine the remaining oil, carrots, zucchini, remaining 1 teaspoon of garlic powder, and the paprika. Season with salt and pepper to taste. Toss to coat. Transfer to a baking sheet.

4   Transfer the baking sheet to the oven, and bake for 10 minutes. Remove from the oven. Flip the vegetables, and make room for the salmon.

5   Place the salmon on the baking sheet with the vegetables, and return it to the oven. Bake for 10 to 13 minutes, or until the salmon flakes easily with a fork and reaches an internal temperature of 145°F. Remove from the oven.

Storage: Keep both the salmon and vegetables in airtight glass containers in the refrigerator for up to 3 days.

Tip: Forgot to thaw your frozen salmon? Just throw it in a bowl of cold running water. It thaws pretty quickly.

Oven-Roasted Drumsticks with Brussels Sprouts

PREP TIME: 10 to 15 minutes **COOK TIME:** 40 to 45 minutes
DAIRY-FREE • **GLUTEN-FREE** • **NUT-FREE**

This yummy one–sheet pan meal makes it easy to cook and clean up. This type of meal is what every parent needs for a busy night, when you can pop it in the oven and walk away to spend time with your family while the oven does the work. **SERVES 6 TO 8**

2 pounds Brussels sprouts, halved

½ onion, thinly sliced

1 tablespoon avocado oil

Juice of ½ lemon

3 tablespoons balsamic vinegar

1 tablespoon maple syrup or honey (if baby is over 12 months old

½ teaspoon kosher salt

½ teaspoon garlic powder

½ teaspoon onion powder

½ teaspoon paprika

¼ teaspoon dried basil

¼ teaspoon dried thyme

¼ teaspoon dried oregano

10 to 12 chicken drumsticks, patted dry

1 Preheat the oven to 425°F. Line a baking sheet with parchment paper.

2 In a large bowl, combine the Brussels sprouts, onion, avocado oil, lemon juice, vinegar, and maple syrup. Toss to coat. Transfer to the prepared baking sheet.

3 In a small bowl, to make the spice blend, combine the salt, garlic powder, onion powder, paprika, basil, thyme, and oregano.

4 Season the chicken with the spice blend. Arrange on top of the Brussels sprouts.

5 Transfer the baking sheet to the oven, and roast for 40 to 45 minutes, or until the thickest drumstick reaches an internal temperature of 165°F. Remove from the oven.

Storage: Keep in an airtight glass container in the refrigerator for up to 3 days.

Tip: You could substitute chicken thighs for drumsticks.

Curry Smash Burgers

PREP TIME: 15 to 20 minutes **COOK TIME:** 10 to 25 minutes
NUT-FREE

These curry smash burgers are tasty and thin, making them easy for little hands to pick up. The addition of curry powder yields some new flavors and nutritional benefits, like digestion- and immunity-boosting gains. These burgers are fun as sliders on either whole-wheat (preferably sprouted) buns or lettuce buns. **MAKES 8 TO 10 SMASH BURGERS**

1 pound grass-fed ground beef

1 tablespoon yellow curry powder

1 teaspoon kosher salt

1 teaspoon freshly ground black pepper

1 teaspoon onion powder

1 teaspoon garlic powder

Toppings of choice, such as lettuce, mustard, ketchup, homemade Mayonnaise (page 200), pickles, cheese, sauerkraut; sliced onion, tomato, or avocado

Whole-wheat buns of choice or butter lettuce for wraps

1 In a large bowl, mix together the beef, curry powder, salt, pepper, onion powder, and garlic powder. Form into 8 to 10 small balls.

2 Heat a skillet over medium heat. Flatten the balls into patties with your palms, and put 2 to 3 in the skillet at a time. Cook for 1 to 3 minutes on each side, or until cooked to your desired doneness. Remove from the heat. Serve with your favorite toppings, either wrapped in lettuce or on a bun.

Storage: Keep in an airtight glass container in the refrigerator for up to 3 days.

Sesame Beef Rice Bowl

PREP TIME: 5 minutes, plus at least a few hours to marinate **COOK TIME:** 10 to 15 minutes
FREEZER-FRIENDLY · **DAIRY-FREE** · **GLUTEN-FREE OPTION** · **NUT-FREE**

This Asian-inspired dish checks both the boxes I aim for: nourishing and toddler-approved. Soaking the rice enhances digestion (see Grains, Beans, and Legumes Prep, page 36), and the sesame seeds contain a bit of everything, including antioxidants and minerals such as zinc and fiber. The combination of savory soy sauce, sesame oil, garlic, and scallions brings added flavor to this savory dish. **MAKES ABOUT 6 CUPS**

½ cup low-sodium soy sauce

2 tablespoons toasted sesame oil

2 tablespoons sesame seeds, plus more for garnish

1 tablespoon minced garlic

1 bunch of scallions (white and green parts), chopped

1 pound grass-fed ground beef

Warm rice, for serving

Sauerkraut or kimchi, for serving

1 In a large bowl, mix together the soy sauce, sesame oil, sesame seeds, garlic, scallions, and beef. Refrigerate for a few hours or up to overnight.

2 Heat a medium saucepan over medium-high heat.

3 Add the beef mixture. Cook for 10 to 15 minutes, or until the beef is cooked through and no longer pink. Remove from the heat. Serve over warm rice, topped with sauerkraut.

4 Garnish with sesame seeds.

Storage: Keep in an airtight glass container in the refrigerator for up to 3 days.

Tip: This recipe still tastes great even if you skip marinating the beef. For a gluten-free option, you can use tamari or coconut aminos instead of soy sauce.

Coconut Beef Stroganoff with Mushrooms

PREP TIME: 10 minutes **COOK TIME:** 15 to 20 minutes
FREEZER-FRIENDLY · **DAIRY-FREE** · **NUT-FREE**

Beef stroganoff makes me nostalgic about my childhood. This recipe is a spin-off from the one I grew up eating, and it includes a creamy sauce with coconut milk. **SERVES 4 TO 6**

1 (8-ounce) box of bowtie pasta

1 ½ pounds grass-fed ground beef

2 cups mushrooms, sliced

1 large sweet onion, diced

½ teaspoon kosher salt, or to taste

¼ teaspoon freshly ground black pepper, or to taste

2 cups beef or chicken bone broth

2 tablespoons Dijon mustard

1 tablespoon Worcestershire sauce

1 (15-ounce) can full-fat coconut milk

2 tablespoons oat flour

1 tablespoon cornstarch

Chopped fresh parsley, for garnish (optional)

1   Cook the noodles according to the package directions. Drain.

2   Meanwhile, heat a large skillet over medium-high heat.

3   Put the beef in the skillet. Cook, breaking up the meat, for 2 minutes, or until browned. Transfer to a plate.

4   Add the mushrooms, onion, salt and pepper to the skillet. Sauté for about 5 minutes, or until the onion is soft.

5   Add the bone broth, mustard, and Worcestershire sauce.

6   In a small bowl, whisk together the coconut milk, flour, and cornstarch. Whisk into the skillet.

7   Return the beef to the skillet, and simmer for about 3 minutes until cooked through. Remove from the heat.

8   Put the pasta in a large serving dish. Pour in the stroganoff, and sitr to coat the pasta evenly. Season with salt and pepper to taste. Garnish with parsley (if using).

Storage: Keep in an airtight glass container in the refrigerator for up to 3 days.

Tip: We like to use gluten-free chickpea or lentil noodles, but you could use a whole-wheat bowtie noodle, too.

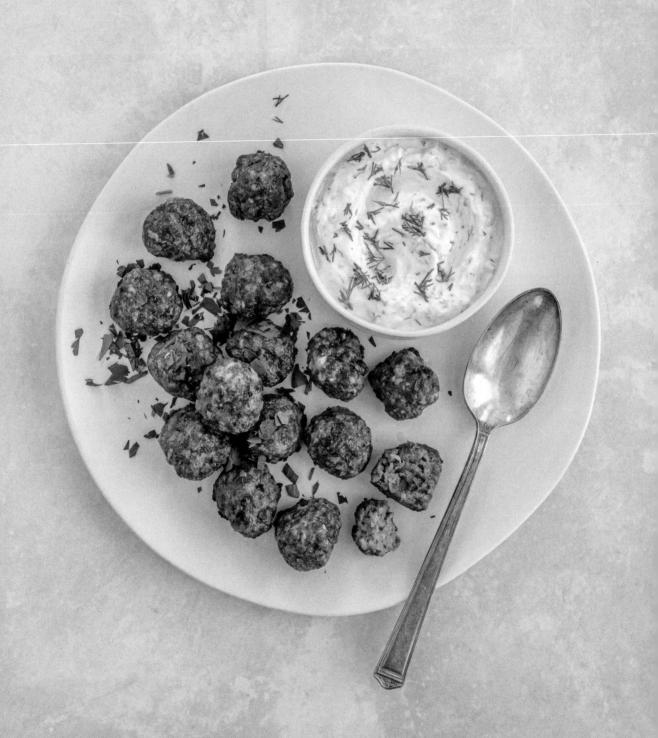

Lamb Meatballs
with Tzatziki Dipping Sauce

PREP TIME: 25 to 35 minutes **COOK TIME:** 20 minutes
NUT-FREE

These little meatballs are great for small hands, and a dip is a fun way to introduce new flavors and textures to your kids. Lamb is a super source of carnitine, an amino acid that moves fatty acids from the bloodstream into the mitochondria (our cells' powerhouses) so the body can use them for energy. The tzatziki sauce is best made ahead of time and left in the refrigerator to let the flavors meld together. **MAKES 16 MEATBALLS**

FOR THE TZATZIKI SAUCE:

½ large English cucumber

1 ½ cups plain, full-fat Greek yogurt

2 teaspoons minced garlic

2 tablespoons extra-virgin olive oil

1 tablespoon white vinegar

½ teaspoon kosher salt

1 tablespoon minced fresh dill

FOR THE MEATBALLS:

1 pound grass-fed ground lamb

1 large egg

½ cup panko bread crumbs

1 tablespoon minced garlic

2 tablespoons chopped fresh parsley

2 tablespoons chopped fresh oregano

1 teaspoon ground cumin

1 teaspoon kosher salt

½ teaspoon freshly ground black pepper

¼ teaspoon red pepper flakes (optional)

3 tablespoons olive oil

TO MAKE THE TZATZIKI SAUCE:

1 Grate the cucumber, and drain through a thin cotton dishcloth to remove excess liquid. Wring out the cucumber to remove maximum moisture. If you don't have a thin cotton dish towel, just squeeze out as much liquid as you can with your hands.

2 In a medium bowl, combine the cucumber, yogurt, garlic, olive oil, vinegar, and salt.

3 Add the dill. Refrigerate while you make the meatballs. ➥

TO MAKE THE MEATBALLS:

1 Preheat the oven to 425°F. Line a baking sheet with parchment paper.

2 In a large bowl, with clean hands, combine the lamb, egg, bread crumbs, garlic, parsley, oregano, cumin, salt, pepper, and red pepper flakes (if using). Roll and form into 16 meatballs. Transfer to the prepared baking sheet.

3 Drizzle with the olive oil.

4 Transfer the baking sheet to the oven, and bake for 20 minutes, or until golden and cooked through. Remove from the oven. Serve warm with the tzatziki sauce.

Storage: Keep the sauce and meatballs in separate airtight glass containers in the refrigerator for up to 3 days.

Tip: If you don't have a grater, just finely chop the cucumber. You can substitute ground beef for lamb. Leftover tzatziki is great with rye bread and naan and works well as a dip for raw veggies.

Quiche Lorraine with Sweet Potato Crust

PREP TIME: 15 to 20 minutes **COOK TIME:** 1 hour
FREEZER-FRIENDLY · **GLUTEN-FREE** · **NUT-FREE**

This quiche satisfies all my favorite breakfast requirements: non-starchy veggies, protein, and sweet potatoes. Of course, it makes a delicious lunch or dinner, too. I love to make it once a week in the evening, ensuring that my family can enjoy a quick and nutritious meal for a few days in a row. **SERVES 8**

2 tablespoons coconut oil, for greasing

1 large or 2 small sweet potatoes, peeled and thinly sliced

¼ pound nitrate-free, antibiotic-free deli ham, chopped

1 cup shredded raw Cheddar cheese (optional)

1 cup mushrooms, diced

½ red bell pepper, cored and diced

10 large eggs

1 teaspoon kosher salt

1 teaspoon freshly ground black pepper

1 teaspoon garlic powder

1 teaspoon onion powder

2 cups heavy cream or raw milk or 1 cup coconut cream

1   Preheat the oven to 375°F. Grease 9 x 13-inch baking dish or 2 quiche dishes.

2   Place the sweet potatoes in the baking dish to form a crust, overlapping them well because they will shrink.

3   Transfer the baking dish to the oven, and bake for 20 minutes. Remove from the oven, leaving the oven on.

4   Place the ham and cheese (if using) on top of the sweet potato crust.

5   Place the mushrooms and bell pepper on top of the ham.

6   In a large bowl, beat together the eggs, salt, pepper, garlic powder, onion powder, and heavy cream. Pour over the crust.

7   Return the baking dish to the oven, and bake for about 40 minutes. Remove from the oven. Let stand for 5 to 10 minutes before slicing.

Storage: Keep in an airtight glass container in the refrigerator for up to 4 days.

Tip: You could also make this with baking potatoes.

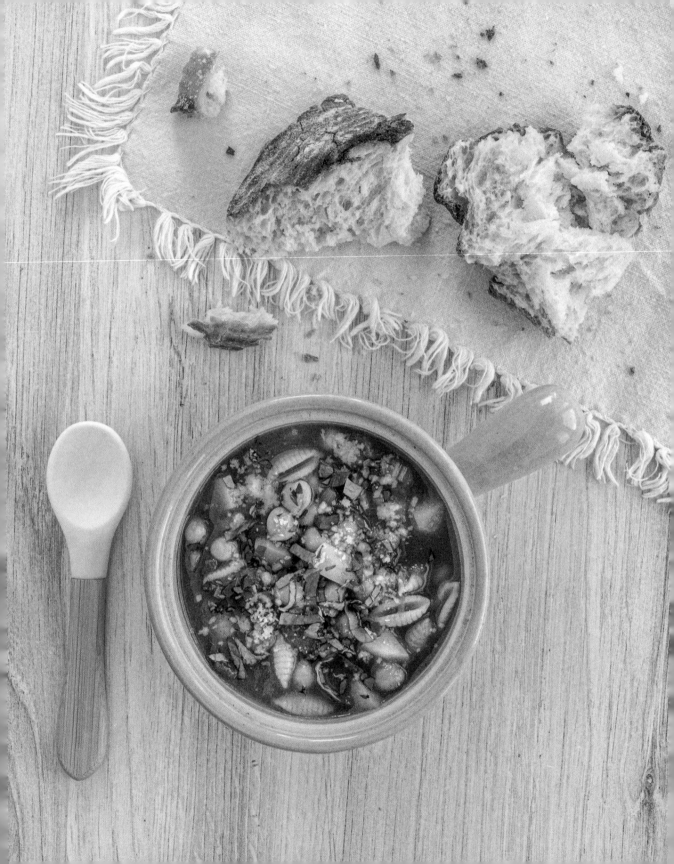

Chickpea Minestrone Soup

PREP TIME: 20 minutes, plus overnight to soak the chickpeas COOK TIME: 30 to 35 minutes
FREEZER-FRIENDLY · NUT-FREE · VEGETARIAN OPTION

This nourishing bowl is inspired by the food of Sardinia, Italy. Sardinians are some of the happiest and healthiest people on the planet, and they regularly consume a minestrone similar to this one. Join in the health and happiness by eating the rainbow in a form the whole family will enjoy!

MAKES ABOUT 4 QUARTS

2 cups dried chickpeas

½ tablespoon apple cider vinegar

Warm filtered water

3 tablespoons olive oil

1 medium yellow or white onion, chopped

2 carrots, chopped

2 celery stalks, chopped

1 tablespoon minced garlic

1 (28-ounce) can diced tomatoes

3 medium yellow potatoes, peeled and diced (about 1 ½ cups)

1 ½ to 2 quarts bone broth or filtered water

1 cup macaroni pasta

Kosher salt and freshly ground black pepper to taste

Chopped fresh basil and parsley, for garnish

Freshly grated Parmesan or Romano cheese, for garnish

1. Put the chickpeas and vinegar in a large bowl. Cover with warm filtered water, and let soak overnight. Drain and rinse well.

2. In a large soup pot, heat the olive oil over medium-high heat.

3. Add the onion, carrots, and celery. Cook, stirring, for about 5 minutes, or until they begin to soften.

4. Add the garlic, and cook for about 30 seconds.

5. Add the tomatoes, potatoes, chickpeas, and bone broth, making sure everything is covered by about 1 inch of liquid.

6. Raise the heat to high. Bring to a boil. Cook for 5 to 10 minutes, or until the potatoes and carrots are tender. ➤→

MAINS

7   Stir in the noodles, and cook according to the package directions. Add more liquid if you need to thin out the soup. Season with salt and pepper to taste. Remove from the heat.

8   Garnish with basil, parsley, and cheese. Serve with sourdough bread, if desired.

Storage: Keep in an airtight glass container in the refrigerator for up to 5 days, or freeze for up to 3 months.

Tip: You could use canned chickpeas instead; even soaking canned beans or chickpeas for an hour before cooking can help to unlock more nutrients and break down any phytic acid. You can substitute other beans, or add even more. Pinto, navy, or fava beans are good alternatives. Other seasonal vegetables also make good substitutes; try broccoli, cauliflower, cabbage, green beans or zucchini.

12 TO 18+ MONTHS

Pasta with Chicken and Veggie Marinara

PREP TIME: 15 to 20 minutes **COOK TIME:** 10 to 15 minutes
FREEZER-FRIENDLY • **NUT-FREE**

Although I am a big fan of introducing vegetables in a formal way, there's nothing wrong with disguising them in other foods to enhance a meal. This dish pairs pasta with my blended veggie sauce and added chicken, a perfect well-rounded meal. See Tip for fun-shaped pasta ideas. **SERVES 4 TO 6**

1 (8-ounce) box of pasta (see Tip)

6 to 8 cups bone broth

1 recipe Veggie Marinara (page 160)

1 cup chopped cooked chicken

Freshly grated Parmesan cheese, for topping

1 In a large pot, cook the noodles in the bone broth according to the package directions. Strain the pasta and save the broth for another use. Return the pasta to the pot, add the marinara, toss together, mix in the chicken, and stir to combine.

2 Sprinkle with Parmesan cheese before serving.

Storage: Once cooled, keep leftover marinara in large glass jars, leaving 1 inch at the top, and freeze for up to 3 months.

Tip: Great pasta shapes for toddlers include rotini, bowties, cavatappi, shells, and rotelle.

MAINS

Black Bean Enchiladas with Spinach and Cheese

PREP TIME: 20 minutes **COOK TIME:** 40 minutes
GLUTEN-FREE · **NUT-FREE** · **VEGETARIAN**

This easy casserole is perfect to make a couple days in advance or bake right after you make it. Although there appear to be a lot of steps, it's mostly just layering the ingredients. It's one of my family's favorite meals, The kids always ask for seconds, and it still makes enough to guarantee leftovers!

SERVES 12

1 tablespoon grass-fed, unsalted butter

1 (5-ounce) container baby spinach

2 (15-ounce) cans black beans, drained and rinsed

1 (4-ounce) can green chilies, drained

1 teaspoon ground cumin

1 (16-ounce) jar salsa, any style

12 small sprouted corn tortillas

1 (4-ounce) package goat cheese

2 cups shredded Cheddar cheese

1 ripe avocado, halved, pitted, peeled, and sliced

1 Preheat the oven to 400°F. Have a 9 x 13-in baking dish ready to use.

2 In a skillet, melt the butter over medium heat.

3 Add the spinach, and cook for 2 to 3 minutes, or until wilted. Remove from the heat.

4 In a large bowl, mix together the beans, chilies, and cumin.

5 Pour one third of the salsa into the baking dish.

6 Layer 6 tortillas on top, staggering them.

7 Pour one third of the salsa over the tortillas.

8   Layer the spinach evenly in the baking dish. Add the bean mixture, spreading it evenly.

9   Crumble the goat cheese on top of the beans, and top with the remaining 6 tortillas.

10 Pour in the remaining third of the salsa, and top with the Cheddar cheese. Cover the baking dish with aluminum foil.

11 Transfer the baking dish to the oven, and bake for 20 minutes.

12 Remove the foil, and bake for 15 minutes, or until the cheese is bubbly. Remove from the oven. The enchiladas will seem to have too much liquid while they're still hot. Once the dish cools off, the salsa will set up, and it will be easy to slice.

13 Top with the avocado.

Storage: Keep in an airtight glass container in the refrigerator for up to 3 days.

One-Pot Mushroom and Zucchini Pasta

PREP TIME: 15 to 20 minutes **COOK TIME:** 10 to 15 minutes
DAIRY-FREE OPTION · NUT-FREE

One-pot meals make dinner so simple. This delicious pasta will satisfy your craving for an easy, hearty, and creamy meal, especially on a cold or rainy day, as it fills the house with tempting aromas and fills bellies with warmth and goodness. **SERVES 6**

4 ½ cups bone broth or filtered water

1 pound spaghetti

1 pound cremini mushrooms, sliced

2 small zucchini or yellow squash, thinly sliced and quartered

⅔ cup frozen peas

2 teaspoons minced garlic

2 teaspoons fresh thyme leaves or ½ teaspoon dried

¼ cup heavy cream

⅓ cup grated Parmesan cheese (optional)

Kosher salt and freshly ground black pepper to taste

1   In a large pot, bring the bone broth to a boil. Add the spaghetti, mushrooms, zucchini, peas, garlic, and thyme. Reduce the heat to a simmer. Cook for 8 to 10 minutes, or until the spaghetti is cooked. Remove from the heat.

2   Stir in the heavy cream and Parmesan (if using). Season with salt and pepper to taste.

3   Serve in a bowl.

Storage: Keep in an airtight glass container in the refrigerator for up to 3 days.

Tip: For a dairy-free option, substitute canned coconut milk for the heavy cream. You could replace zucchini with any quick-cooking vegetables, such as broccoli, cauliflower, or spinach.

PICKY EATING

Most parents experience picky eating with their child at some point, often around age 2. I often hear parents say, "Our baby used to eat anything, but is so picky now," as their babies become choosier as toddlers. This is a normal phase, so try not to make a big deal of it, and rest assured it will pass with the help of some of these tips:

OFFER NEW FOODS OR A NEW FORM OF THE FOOD. We can get in the habit of serving their favorite foods to the point of burnout. So, for example, if your toddler rejects once-loved bananas or avocados, try a banana smoothie or guacamole.

SERVE NEW FOODS WITH A WELL-LOVED FOOD. Combining new foods with a food you know they do enjoy can help open their palates to this new flavor.

EAT AS A FAMILY. Once your child is eating the same food as you, make sure they see that you're eating your vegetables, too. It makes sense to nourish yourself the way you are nourishing them. And that means you deserve time to sit down and enjoy your food, too.

DECONSTRUCT THE FOOD. Toddlers like to see everything in their own element so they can further inspect and choose what they want to eat. You can break down a meal and offer things as single ingredients alongside each other. Soups, stews, bowls, and quesadillas are just as nutritious if you offer the ingredients side by side.

DON'T FORCE THEM TO EAT. You're not always in the mood for peas and chicken, so try to be understanding if they aren't in the mood, either. I like to offer an alternate food that I know they'll eat. We don't encourage this every day, but try to understand that they won't always like the food or want to eat what is served.

REINTRODUCE REJECTED FOODS OVER AND OVER AGAIN. Your little one will likely refuse a food several times and then eventually try it. They may really like it one day, so be sure to keep introducing these foods. If you stop serving it altogether, it may never be tried. Taste buds change and so do kids' outlook on trying new foods.

Resources

Baby and Kid Kitchen Gear Brands

- **Avanchy®** (plates and cutlery)
- **Bumkins®** (plates)
- **EzPz™** (cups and spoons)
- **Hydro Flask®** (stainless-steel straw lid water bottle)
- **Philips Avent** (glass bottles)
- **Tovla & Company™** (kid-safe knives and cutting board)
- **Guidecraft®** (kitchen helper stool)

Books

Super Nutrition for Babies by Katherine Erlich and Kelly Genzlinger

The Nourishing Traditions Cookbook for Children by Sally Fallon Morell and Suzanne Gross

Wild Fermentation by Sandor Ellix Katz

Gut and Psychology Syndrome: Natural Treatment for Autism, Dyspraxia, A.D.D., Dyslexia, A.D.H.D., Depression, Schizophrenia by Natasha Campbell-McBride

Nourishing Traditions: Book of Baby & Child Care by Sally Fallon Morell

Real Food for Mother and Baby: The Fertility Diet, Eating for Two, and Baby's First Foods by Nina Planck

Baby-Led Weaning: The Essential Guide to Introducing Solid Food—and Helping Your Baby to Grow Up a Happy and Confident Eater by Gill Rapley and Tracey Murkett

Cod Liver Oil Brands for Kids

- Blue Ice®
- Carlson Labs®
- Green Pastures™
- Nordic Naturals™
- Sonne's

Grass-Fed Collagen or Gelatin Brands for Recipes

- Great Lakes®
- Vital Proteins®

Helpful Web Pages

Fish Mercury Chart (FDA)
www.fda.gov/media/102331/download
The FDA's chart of fish and their mercury content, especially as it applies to young children and pregnant and breastfeeding persons.

Food Scores (Environmental Working Group)
www.ewg.org/foodscores
This provides food scores for whole and processed foods based on ingredients, nutrition, and processing concerns.

Eat a Rainbow (Whole Kids Foundation)

www.wholekidsfoundation.org/assets/docu-ments/better-bites-eat-a-rainbow.pdf

This fun chart shows foods across the rainbow and their benefits.

Homemade Baby Formula (Weston A. Price Foundation)

www.westonaprice.org/health-topics/childrens-health/formula-homemade-baby-formula

A homemade alternative to store-bought formula, with easily digestible ingredients mimicking breast milk.

Non-Dairy Homemade Formula (The Healthy Home Economist)

www.thehealthyhomeeconomist.com/video-hypoallergenic-baby-formula

Hypoallergenic recipe for homemade formula.

Websites: Sources and General Information

Blooming Motherhood

www.bloomingmotherhood.co

The author's website, which offers guidance on first foods for littles, emphasis on prevention of allergies and chronic illnesses, and reversing eczema. Teaches modern moms how to integrate ancient and natural medicine into the daily rhythm.

U.S. Wellness Meats

www.grasslandbeef.com

They carry an inventory of quality bones and ship to all 50 states, Puerto Rico, and Canada.

Kelly Mom

www.kellymom.com

Up-to-date and evidence-based information for breastfeeding and parenting.

Lily Nichols, RDN, CDE

www.lilynicholsrdn.com

A real-food approach combining traditional wisdom with modern eating for moms and kids, with emphasis on evidenced-based prenatal nutrition and first foods.

La Leche League International (LLLI)

www.llli.org

They provide breastfeeding information, domestic and global, and assists in finding support for breastfeeding near you.

A Campaign for Real Milk

www. realmilk.com

A good resource for finding real milk near you. It is a project of the Weston A. Price Foundation.

Solid Starts

www. solidstarts.com

The only food database in the world just for babies.

The Weston A. Price Foundation

www. westonaprice.org

An inclusive approach for eating all types of foods, complete with accurate and scientific research, it has multiple articles pertaining to children and babies.

References

A Baby Food Revolution. Last modified, 2020. *https://solidstarts.com/.*

Amarelo, Monica, and Samara Geller. "5 Ways to Reduce Your Exposure to Toxic BPA." EWG. Last modified February 9, 2018. *https://www.ewg.org/news-and-analysis/2018/02/5-ways-reduce-your-exposure-toxic-bpa.*

"Advice About Eating Fish." FDA. Accessed May 16, 2020. *https://www.fda.gov/media/102331/download.*

Bittner, George D., Chun Z. Yang, and Matther A. Stoner. "Estrogenic chemicals often leach from BPA-free plastic products that are replacements for BPA-containing polycarbonate products." *Environmental Health* 31 (May 28, 2014). *https://ehjournal.biomedcentral.com/articles/10.1186/1476-069X-13-41.*

"Breastfeeding Report Card." CDC Centers for Disease Control and Prevention. Last modified, 2014. *https://www.cdc.gov/breastfeeding/pdf/2014breastfeedingreportcard.pdf.*

"Broth is Beautiful." Last modified January 1, 2000. *https://www.westonaprice.org/health-topics/food-features/broth-is-beautiful/.*

"Canaries in the kitchen: tips on safe cookware." EWG. Last modified May 15, 2003. *https://www.ewg.org/research/canaries-kitchen/tips-safe-cookware.*

"Dirty Dozen Endocrine Disruptors 12 Hormone-Altering Chemicals and How to Avoid Them." EWG. Last modified October 28, 2013. *https://www.ewg.org/research/dirty-dozen-list-endocrine-disruptors.*

Du Toit, George, Graham Roberts, Peter H. Sayre, Henry T. Bahnson, and Suzana Radulovic. "Randomized Trial of Peanut Consumption in Infants at Risk for Peanut Allergy." *The New England Journal of Medicine* 372, no. 9 (February 26, 2015): 803-13. *https://doi.org/10.1056/NEJMoa1414850.*

Evivo. Accessed March 2, 2020. *https://www.evivo.com/professionals/infant-gut-microbiome.*

Fallon Morell, Sally, and Hilda L. Gore. "Wise Traditions Podcast Episode #58: Should we eat grains? (Principle 6)." The Weston A. Price Foundation for Wise Traditions in Food, Farming and the Healing Arts. Last modified January 6, 2017. *https://www.westonaprice.org/podcast/58-should-we-eat-grains/.*

Fallon Morell, Sally, and Mary G. Enig, PhD. "Be Kind to Your Grains . . . And Your Grains Will Be Kind To You." The Weston A. Price Foundation for Wise Traditions in Food, Farming and the Healing Arts. Last modified January 1, 2000. *https://www.westonaprice.org/health-topics/food-features/be-kind-to-your-grains-and-your-grains-will-be-kind-to-you/.*

Francino, M.P. "Antibiotics and the Human Gut Microbiome: Dysbioses and Accumulation of Resistances." *Frontiers in Microbiology* 1543, no. 6 (January 12, 2016). *https://doi.org/10.3389/fmicb.2015.01543.*

Gillard, B.K., J.A. Simbala, and L. Goodglick. "Reference Intervals for Amylase Isoenzymes in Serum and Plasma of Infants and Children." *Clinical Chemistry,* 29, no. 6 (1 June 1983) *https://doi.org/10.1093/clinchem/29.6.1119.*

Greer, Frank R., Scott H. Sicherer, and A. Burks. "The Effects of Early Nutritional Interventions on the Development of Atopic Disease in Infants and Children: The Role of Maternal Dietary Restriction, Breastfeeding, Hydrolyzed Formulas, and Timing of." *Pediatrics* 143, no. 4 (April 2019). *https://doi.org/10.1542/peds.2019-0281.*

Hartke, Kimberly. "Government Data Proves Raw Milk Safe." The Weston A. Price Foundation for Wise Traditions in Food, Farming and the Healing Arts. Last modified August 1, 2011. *https://www.westonaprice.org/government-data-proves-raw-milk-safe/.*

Huh, Susanna, Sheryl L. Rifas-Shiman, Elsie M. Tavaras, Emily Oken, and Matthew Gillman. "Timing of Solid Food Introduction and Risk of Obesity in Preschool-Aged Children." *Pediatrics* (March 2011): 127. *https://doi.org/10.1542/peds.2010-0740.*

"Is plastic a threat to your health?" Harvard Health Publishing of Harvard Medical School. Last modified December, 2019. *https://www.health.harvard.edu/staying-healthy/is-plastic-a-threat-to-your-health.*

"Keep Food Safe! Food Safety Basics." USDA FSIS. Last modified December 20, 2016. *https://www.fsis.usda.*

gov/wps/portal/fsis/topics/food-safety-education/ get-answers/food-safety-fact-sheets/safe-food-handling/keep-food-safe-food-safety-basics/ ct_index.

Klein, Amy. "Baby-Led Weaning: Pros, Cons, and Considering A Moderate Approach." Cincinnati Children's. Last modified April 23, 2019. blog.cincinnatichildrens.org/healthy-living/ child-development-and-behavior/baby-led-weaning-pros-cons-and-considering-a-moderate-approach.

Konieczna, Aleksandra, Aleksandra Rutkowska, and Dominik Rachoń. "Health Risk of Exposure to Bisphenol A (BPA)." Rocz Panstw Zakl Hig 66, no. 1: 5–11. Accessed April 1, 2020. https://www.ncbi.nlm. nih.gov/pubmed/25813067.

Lozoff, Betsy, John Beard, James Connor, Barbara Felt, and Michael Georgieff. "Long-Lasting Neural and Behavioral Effects of Iron Deficiency in Infancy." Nutrition Reviews 64, no. 5 (August 14, 2006). https:// www.ncbi.nlm.nih.gov/pmc/articles/PMC1540447.

"Mercury Levels in Commercial Fish and Shellfish (1990-2012)." FDA. Last modified October 25, 2017. https://www.fda.gov/food/metals-and-your-food/ mercury-levels-commercial-fish-and-shellfish-1990-2012.

Michaelis CNC, Kristen. "Why ditch the infant cereals?" food renegade. Last modified June 25, 2019. https://www.foodrenegade.com/ why-ditch-infant-cereals/.

Mnif, Wissem, Aziza Hadj Hassine, Aicha Bouaziz, Aghleb Bartegi, and Olivier Thomas. "Effect of Endocrine Disruptor Pesticides: A Review." International Journal of Res Public Health 8, no. 6 (June 17, 2011): 2265-303. https://doi.org/10.3390/ ijerph8062265.

"National Center for Health Statistics." CDC Centers for Disease Control and Prevention. Last modified, 2018. Accessed May 6, 2020. https://www.cdc.gov/nchs/ fastats/delivery.htm.

Neuman, Hadar, Paul Forsythe, Atara Uzan, Orly Avni, and Omry Koren. "Antibiotics in early life: dysbiosis and the damage done." FEMS Microbiology Reviews 42, no. 4 (July 25, 2018): 439-99. https://doi. org/10.1093/femsre/fuy018.

Otsuki, M., H. Yuu, S. Saeki, and S. Baba. "The Characteristics of Amylase Activity and the Isoamylase Pattern in Serum and Urine of Infants and Children." European Journal of Pediatrics (July 1, 1977): 175-80. https://doi.org/10.1007/BF00480594.

"Perfluorooctanoic Acid (PFOA), Teflon, and Related Chemicals." Cancer.org. Last modified March 4, 2020. https://www.cancer.org/cancer/cancer-causes/ teflon-and-perfluorooctanoic-acid-pfoa.html.

Prado, Elizabeth L., and Kathryn G. Dewey. "Nutrition and Brain Development in Early Life." Nutrition Reviews 72, no. 4 (April 2014). https://doi.org/10.1111/ nure.12102.

Russo, Pasquale, Paloma Lopez, Vittorio Capozzi, Pilar Fernandez de Palencia, and Maria Teresa Duenas. Beta-glucans Improve Growth, Viability and Colonization of Probiotic Microorganisms." International Journal of Molecular Sciences 13, no. 5 (May 18, 2012): 6026-39. https://doi.org/10.3390/ ijms13056026.

Sears, Dr. William. Ask Dr. Sears: The Trusted Resource for Parents. Last modified, May 1, 2020. https://www. askdrsears.com/.

Sicherer, MD, Scott, and Frank R. Greer, MD. "Dietary interventions to prevent atopic disease: Updated recommendations." AAP NEWS. Last modified March 18, 2019. https://www.aappublications.org/ news/2019/03/18/atopy031819.

Siebecker, Allison. "Traditional Bone Broth in Modern Health and Disease." Townsend Letter, the Examiner of Alternative Medicine/Townsend Letter for Doctors & Patients (March 2005). https://www. townsendletter.com/FebMarch2005/broth0205.htm.

Tye, J.G., R.C. Karn, and A.D. Merritt. "Differential expression of salivary (Amy1) and pancreatic (Amy2) human amylase loci in prenatal and postnatal development." Journal of Medical Genetics (April 13, 1976): 96–102. https://doi.org/10.1136/jmg.13.2.96.

Weidenhamer, Jeffrey, Meghann P. Fitzpatrick, Alison M. Biro, Peter A. Kobunski, and Michael R. Hudson. "Metal Exposures From Aluminum Cookware: An Unrecognized Public Health Risk in Developing Countries." Science of the Total Environment 579 (February 1, 2017): 805–13. https://doi. org/10.1016/j.scitotenv.2016.11.023.

Young Yoon, Mi, and Sang Sun Yoon. "Disruption of the Gut Ecosystem by Antibiotics." Yonsei Medical Journal 50, no. 1 (November 29, 2017): 4–12. https:// doi.org/10.3349/ymj.2018.59.1.4.

Recipe Index

Index

Acknowledgments

Thank you, Elowen and Aldrik. Without you, I would not be a mother and I may have never fallen into my calling for nourishing littles. Thank you for teaching me how resilient kids are. You are love, joy, peace, and light. I love you.

Thank you, Trenton, for every dish you cleaned behind me, for helping me in the kitchen while I whirled around making messes, for taking the kids on long adventures so I could recipe-test, and for your commitment to nourishing our children together. There were many late nights you stayed up with me—your honesty and support is unmatched.

Thank you to my parents, who instilled in me the importance and love of real food. Thank you, Mom, for growing fresh herbs in the kitchen all year and saying "no" to aspartame before it was cool to do so. Thank you, Dad, for befriending local farmers and showing us resources for growing our own food. You've both so positively impacted how I nourish my body.

Thank you to my friends who supported me during the writing period. Alex Maurer, Leanna Ward, Julianna Campbell, Allee Mixon, Madison Morrigan, Karisa Cook, Susanna Depriest, and Kinsey Olson: thank you for offering your kids as honest taste testers, continuously encouraging me, and for working and mothering alongside me. I am forever grateful for our friendships.

Thank you Megan Mixon for loving on my children as I wrote the book. Thank you for making my home look like there was never a tornado of toys after a long day of writing, and for lighting up my children's imaginations.

Thank you to my family and friends who tested and tasted. A special thanks to my dad, my Aunt Katherine, my cousin Joseph Bodenbach, and Chelcea Burns. Thank you to my clients who volunteered their time to test recipes alongside me and included their adventurous and cute children as taste testers. You've all elevated my cooking and recipes with your expertise.

Thank you to all of my clients, past and current, for trusting me and giving me the opportunity to live out my dream of being a nurse. You are all are the reason I keep documenting my kitchen, my food, and my kids.

Thank you to some of my dearest and oldest friends: Lauren Maness, thank you for embarking on a "health" journey with me over a decade ago, and for offering your dietician intelligence and wisdom as I wrote this book. Kelli Randall, thank you for sharing in our life's biggest enthusiasms, from babies to books.

Thank you to my editor, Meg Ilasco, for seeing my potential, answering all my questions, and for making this book come together. I looked forward to each conversation and I am forever grateful for your guidance, kindness, and expertise throughout this process.

Thank you to everyone on the Zeitgeist Team at Penguin Random House who helped me so much in the book's creation including Shara Beitch and Katy Brown. Special thanks to Nancy Cho for such beautiful photos and to editors Will, Patty, Valerie, and Mary for your expert attention to detail and wisdom in food and editing.

About the Author

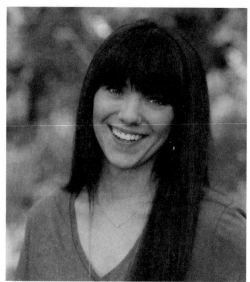

Joe Camden

Leah Bodenbach, RN, BSN, is a nurse, coach, and founder of Blooming Motherhood. After receiving her nursing degree in 2014, she worked in a hospital setting in neuro trauma, pediatric ICU, neonatal ICU, and postpartum. Simultaneously, she worked at a birthing center, assisting midwives in supporting moms and babies through natural labor and childbirth.

She now specializes in reducing the risk of allergies and chronic health issues through first foods for littles. She is wildly passionate about teaching moms to nourish their little ones with intentional foods, as well as how to integrate holistic and modern medicine into their own daily rhythm.

Leah resides in Springfield, Missouri, with her husband, Trenton, and their two children, Elowen and Aldrik. She loves relaxing in a hammock, working in her garden with her husband, cooking with her kids, dancing around the house, and hearing live music. You can sign up to work one-on-one with Leah at *bloomingmotherhood.co* for an individualized approach to first foods, or an integrative approach to wellness for your little one.